COUNSELLING in NURSING

A Problem-Solving Approach

William Stewart, BA, SRN, RMN, DipSocStud

Senior Nursing Officer (Allocation)
Southampton University Hospitals
Combined School of Nursing

Foreword by Annie T Altschul
Emeritus Professor of Nursing Studies
University of Edinburgh

Harper & Row, Publishers
London

Cambridge
Mexico City
New York
Philadelphia

San Francisco
São Paulo
Singapore
Sydney

First published 1983
Reprinted 1986, 1987

Harper & Row Ltd
28 Tavistock Street
London WC2E 7PN

British Library Cataloguing in Publication Data

Stewart, William
   Counselling in nursing
   1. Nursing—Great Britain
   2. Counselling—Great Britain
   I. Title
   362.1′04256   RT42

ISBN 0-06-318259-9

Typeset by Activity, Salisbury, Wilts
Printed by Butler and Tanner Ltd, Frome and London

To Margaret

CONTENTS

Appendices

FOREWORD

Over the past few years more and more nurses have been heard to refer to their role in counselling. Many have expressed a need for training in this activity, some have shown concern about the responsibility thrust upon them.

In so far as progress has been made in the dissemination of interest and skill, the author is entitled to claim a large share of the credit for it. His writings on the subject have been well received. His own experience as a nurse and a counsellor entitles him to write with authority. He has a knack of addressing his readership in a direct way, on a basis of equality. He credits his readers with knowledge, experience and a high degree of motivation. He assumes that he shares with his readers the conceptual framework of counselling, namely, that of a relationship within which a person in need of help can explore alternative ways of coping with a problem. It is pleasant to see the concept of counselling used in this wholly appropriate way, and not, as is so often the case, misused as a synonym for criticism and disciplinary action.

In this book the author goes further than in his earlier writing in explaining what he means by counselling. He describes a method which is akin to the social worker's or the psychotherapist's process of establishing and using relationships. The parallel between the model of counselling and that of the nursing process is clearly demonstrated.

Traditionally much of what is valuable in nursing is in direct conflict with the ethos of counselling. Nurses value decisiveness, giving directives, getting quick results, taking charge of situations, suppressing troublesome feelings.

Counselling is a method of withholding advice, refraining from decisionmaking, exploring feelings, leading the client to the discovery of his own coping mechanism. Counselling skills do not come naturally to nurses. This book will help them to learn them.

The text is liberally illustrated with snippets of case studies which amply exemplify the principles which are being discussed.

The author is an advocate for the use of the nursing process and a believer in the value of nursing the whole patient. His examples of counselling demonstrate, however, how difficult it would be to draw up a nursing plan for the whole patient and how one can only touch on a very small fraction of the problem of any client.

I am convinced that this book will fill an urgent need of nurses at every level of their careers. Every nurse's relationships with patients and others will be enhanced by the understanding developed through studying this book.

Annie T. Altschul
Emeritus Professor of Nursing Studies
University of Edinburgh
1983

PREFACE

This book was conceived in Holland in April 1979, when I attended the Second International Congress on Patient Counselling and Education.* As I listened to the many speakers, and the subsequent discussion, I realized, possibly more clearly than ever before, just how many nurses there were, in all parts of the world, actively involved in counselling patients.

One area particularly caught my attention and imagination: the rights of the patient. When one considers the rights of the patient, one must also consider the rights and responsibilities of those who care for him. One of the patient's rights (which is discussed later) is to receive, or not to receive—if he so wishes—information related to his condition and treatment. One of the rights of those who care for patients is to be given adequate training. Clinical training is outside the scope of this book. The area on which I have chosen to concentrate, therefore, is the need for nurses to develop counselling skills.

Though I have chosen to write to nurses, a great deal of the content is pertinent to all who are involved in caring for others. Of all those who have contact with the patient, it is probably the nurse who has the opportunity to spend the most time with him.

The nurse's role is diverse, and nurses practise in a variety of different areas, each of which may present its own problems and difficulties—for the patient and for the nurse. The premise on which this book is written, is that the skills acquired in counselling training have a direct bearing on the nurse's approach to her central role of patient care.

This book does not advocate that nurses need to become professional counsellors. Rather, it suggests that counselling training and practice

---

*Organized by Excerpta Medica Foundation.

should provide some understanding of what is involved; to help achieve some insight and an appreciation of counselling, in order to provide First Aid counselling cover. It is not intended to undervalue or underestimate professional counsellors or what they do, any more than those who train First Aiders undervalue or underestimate doctors and nurses. The one complements, but does not replace, the other.

Nurses cannot help but be drawn into counselling. The very nature of the job demands it, particularly when they are involved in the nursing process. This book endeavours to show how nurses may acquire and use counselling skills for the benefit of the patient, his relatives, the organization and to further their own professional development. If nurses develop more understanding of themselves, their patients and their colleagues, their working environments will become healthier places in which to work.

Nurses—particularly learners, who move frequently—may ask, "Should I start counselling a patient when I'm soon to move to another ward?" This is a dilemma; for rightly, there would be little time or opportunity to develop a relationship with the patient. Having said this, though, the fact that a patient is admitted does not prevent a nurse carrying out whatever nursing treatment is appropriate, even if it is her last day on that ward. The treatment which she started will be carried on by others.

While it is true that the quality of the counselling relationship is influenced by the frequency of contact, much can be achieved within a single session. Just as the nurse, using the nursing process, begins the assessment stage, then hands over to another nurse to continue, so one nurse may begin the counselling process. She would, of course, make sure that the patient understands that someone else will have to continue. This may limit the extent to which the patient is prepared to commit himself, but far better this than for the patient to unburden himself and not have the opportunity to explore what he has disclosed. Sensitively handled, the nurse can safely remove herself from the horns of the dilemma to the benefit of all concerned.

The extent to which nurses are helped to acquire and develop counselling skills depends, to a great extent, on the commitment, encouragement and the example of senior nurses, in all spheres of work.

William Stewart
Bishopstoke, 1983

PART I

THE PROCESS

CHAPTER 1

PATIENT COUNSELLING

What is patient counselling?

Patient counselling is "helping the patient to cope with his condition and the treatment involved". A linked idea is 'patient education', which is "helping the patient to understand and handle his condition and the treatment involved".* It would be useful to examine both of these statements simultaneously for they are so interrelated that they cannot stand independent of each other.

Involving the patient

Patients may not always be involved in the decisions which are taken concerning their treatment. The patient may be told, "take these, three times a day"; and by a process of deduction he will assume that people with his condition always have two red pills and one tiny white one. But this is not true understanding. Most nurses will be able to recall at least one incident where the patient has refused to take his prescribed treatment. Sometimes explanations are given but quite often they are not. This can be bewildering to the patient and to the nursing staff. One such patient was Harry.

Harry was in a medical ward, suffering from a severe respiratory disease for which he had been prescribed some very costly antibiotic capsules. On about the fourth day there was puzzlement because of his nonresponse to treatment. When the nurses were making his bed, his handkerchief dropped out of his pyjama pocket and in it ... 16 large yellow capsules! The nurses told the doctor; the doctor told the consultant and the consultant—well! I'm not sure who he told, but it seemed that everyone was there, gathered round Harry's bed, like a terrifying inquisition. "Do you realize how much these cost?" said one. "Do you want to get better?" said another. Sister castigated the nurses (sotto voce, of course, but still loud enough for at least one of the doctors to hear). When the 'trial' was over (not that Harry said anything, he was too overwhelmed) the retinue swept into the sister's office for another session.

At the 'post mortem' the medical staff tended to blame the nurses, that they had not been vigilant enough. But all the nurses who administered the medicines were convinced that Harry had taken the capsules.

---

*Both of these statement are taken from the programme of the Second International Congress on Patient Counselling and Education held at the Hague in May 1979.

Edward, a mature pupil nurse who had recently been allocated to that particular ward, had an interesting talk with Harry.

E: Harry, you seem to have caused quite a stir—lots of red faces.
H: I feel pretty bad about it all.
E: Do you; in what way?
H: Well everyone was going on at me. I felt like a criminal. Have I done something so awful?
E: They seem to think so.
H: Do you?
E: Only in as much as it does put the nurses in a bit of a spot.
H: I know. I felt really sorry for them. Sister was nearly in tears.
E: You didn't think it could backfire like this, is that it?
H: No, I suppose not. I just couldn't take these things ...
E: Yes? (Pause)
H: I know this sounds silly, but when I tried to take the first one it got stuck. There wasn't anyone else around. The nurse had given me a drink and then moved on and the blooming thing stuck. It wouldn't come up or go down. I thought I was going to die. When they next came round, I pretended to swallow it, then took it out. I've always been difficult with tablets and things; it seems as if my throat seizes up on me. Can anything be done?
E: I'm sure it can. I'll speak to sister.

This shortened version shows how a few minutes careful listening may help. At no time did Edward ask Harry why he had not taken his medication. When Harry and Edward were on the same wavelength, Harry felt he could trust talking about something that 'sounded silly'. If Harry had been properly involved, this situation may have been avoided.

Effective treatment so often hinges on involving the patient, as the following extract shows.

Joseph, aged 28, was due to come into hospital for a menesectomy operation. When his admission date arrived, he was disappointed to discover that it clashed with his first wedding anniversary. He telephoned the admissions clerk, "Is it possible to rearrange the admission? It's quite important and ..." The clerk cut him short with, "No, that is quite impossible. You must keep the appointment or wait your turn again." Joseph did not attempt to argue, but instead, came up to speak to the sister. By this time he was feeling awkward and guilty that he was making such a fuss. The sister put him at his ease and understood his predicament. She explained how difficult it would be to rearrange the operation and together they looked at an alternative; which was to delay the time of admission so that Joseph and his wife could have lunch together and he would come in afterwards. The surgeon agreed, so everyone was satisfied; except the admissions clerk who complained that she had been made to look silly.

There are many instances where involvement of the patient is vital if he is to understand his condition or perhaps learn to cope with it. Everyday conditions which involve the taking of medication may seem straightforward enough, but, as in the case of Harry, it is not always so. Patients who have to administer their own medication—by any route—often need a great deal of support. Even when the technique—injection of insulin, for instance—has been mastered, emotional difficulties may alter the emotional balance which exists between the prescribed treatment and its administration.

Consider the patient who every day must give himself an injection of insulin. His whole life is geared to this, and, in the words of one person, "Sometimes I feel I just can't stick another needle into myself." A woman suffering from a chronic skin complaint said, "Every day I have to plaster myself with that horrible stuff. Sometimes I want to throw the jar through the window." These situations, in a way, are imposed on these patients by their conditions; but is the woman who takes the contraceptive pill any different? She takes the pill voluntarily, or so it appears. But do some take the pill because they feel pressured by society to conform to a family norm? If this is how they feel, is it possible that they could experience resentment? If they do, perhaps their resentment will be expressed in 'forgetting' to take the pill at the crucial time. Is it possible that, for some, the drive to reproduce is stronger than the pressures of society?

Communicating with patients

There is no formula to ensure that the patient becomes actively involved. Some people think that information will be understood if it is clearly given. It is certainly essential to give information clearly, but understanding by the recipient is vital. One person may say to another, "Do you understand?" and think that if the other says, "Yes, I do", that communication has been effective, resulting in understanding. This is not necessarily so. How many of us, when asked if we understand, will readily admit that we do not? It is necessary, therefore, to make certain that the patient understands, by asking suitable questions; open-ended questions that demand more than a 'yes', 'no' answer. A useful technique is for the nurse to ask the person to explain, in his own words, what he thinks she has been telling him. This allows him to hear what he is saying, which may not be exactly what the message was. Not only does this provide an opportunity for the patient to clarify things in his own mind, it allows the nurse to listen to the emotional undertones. It is the emotions which are most likely to cause difficulty. In other words, emotional acceptance of the message is vital: intellectual acceptance is not sufficient. Intellectual acceptance without emotional acceptance gives rise to what appears to be unwillingness and noncompliance.

John and Mary were both in their late 70s when Mary fell and broke her femur. John, only a short time before this, had slowed down, due to heart failure. Mary was admitted to hospital some 20 miles away which made visiting difficult. Mary's progress was hampered by pressure sores on her heels and when she did get up and about, movement was difficult. She did try to walk with a frame but lacked confidence. John agitated to have his wife home, saying he was well able to cope. When Mary did come home she still had to be aided in her walking. The community nurse tried, on several occasions, to get Mary to use the frame on her own, but she quickly saw that both she and John were fearful. Gradually the nurse came to realize that, even though she might get Mary walking, even without the frame, by persevering, John would have difficulty coping with the anxiety. If Mary, who had always been very independent, could walk, she might very well have a repeat fall. All the time she was kept chair-bound, she needed to be helped by John. All the time she was kept under his watchful eye, he could cope. The nurse had to weigh up all these pros and cons: Would increasing Mary's independence increase John's anxiety and stress above tolerable levels? Would that stress be greater than his failing heart could stand? and Would the stress be greater than the physical strain produced by the constant caring for Mary, a semi-invalid? She talked this over with them—not putting it in such direct terms—and was convinced that Mary, somehow, had lost more than her confidence; some of her drive for independence had gone, and without this it would have been difficult to achieve the mobility which could have created conflict between husband and wife.

This emphasizes that not only is intellectual understanding important—John understood everything that was involved—but emotional commitment is vital; something John appeared to have difficulty coming to terms with.

These examples demonstrate how communication operates at different levels. At one level there are the words and at another, their meanings or what is referred to as the 'deep structures' (Chomsky 1968), which vary enormously.

There are occasions when it is perfectly in order to communicate at a surface or superficial level. A party would be an occasion where it would hardly seem necessary to take too much notice of the underlying meanings. But in the context of communicating with patients, it is necesary to communicate at a different level if they and the nurses are to understand each other. This last phrase is very important. Communication between people is often influenced by how well they know each other. Relationships influence communication.

Most people could think of situations where misunderstandings have arisen due to the tone of voice of the other person, but then someone else who knows that other person better has said, "Oh, that's just her manner, she doesn't mean it." The fact that this may be true is not always imediately apparent. As the relationship deepens, understanding often increases. In a similar way, the more we get to know certain people, the more we realize that they are awkward, all the time and to everyone, and that communication between them and other people is difficult. Misunderstanding and confusion may arise from what is actually said. Some people are not always clear in what they say. Attention has already been drawn to how important it is, when dealing with patients, to establish exactly that they do understand. Words are vehicles for conveying feelings but feelings often prevent one person hearing what the other person intended he should hear.

People who become patients assume a new role in relation to a variety of different people—doctors, paramedicals, nurses and domestic staff. Even the word 'patient' evokes many different emotions. Patients are people who are *ill*, looked after in *hospital* by various *specialists* and given *treatment* for some *disease*. Sometimes the treatment is successful and the patient is *discharged*; sometimes it is unsuccessful and the patient *dies*. A patient may experience emotions attached to any or all of these words; and these emotions may interfere with communication. What he says, and what he hears others say, will be coloured by his emotions. The very words which nurses use as part of their vocabulary may sound strange and frightening. This may seem surprising when one thinks of the number of television and radio programmes which feature hospital life. One would think that the general public would be as familiar with nursing jargon as nurses are. But, in a sense, they have caught only part of the meaning—within the specific context in which it was used—and may not be able to apply it to other contexts.

For much of the time, verbal communication between nurse and patient is at a superficial level and is geared towards giving and receiving information or the exchange of pleasantries. The nurse has many opportunities during a working day to engage in communication at a deeper level. If such communication does not always take place, it could be that it is not actively encouraged by senior staff. It could also be that not everyone has the ability to communicate at this level, but such skills may be learned. It is a sad reflection on their stay in hospital that patients can say, "I was very well cared for, but the only people I could really talk to were the other patients." Nurses are able to make it very plain to patients when their verbal approaches are unwelcome. The way the nurse moves swiftly from bed to bed, giving the impression of controlled haste, is enough to deter most people from trying to establish communication at anything other than a superficial level. It is difficult to talk through a thermometer—a very effective way of stifling an awkward patient's flow of conversation! How difficult it is to converse with a nurse so obviously counting the pulse, or peering intently at a pulsating head of mercury with a stethescope jammed firmly in her ears! Another aspect of communication is that conversation between staff and patients may be kept deliberately superficial by such techniques as joking, laughter and banter and a certain amount of horseplay. These avoidance techniques, which may be unconscious, are a way of ensuring that deeper feelings are not readily available to be discussed.

Physical contact

Not all communication is verbal; body posture, gestures and facial expression all have meaning. An area which is worthy of consideration is what Hall (1959) refers to as the 'ideal sphere'; the territory around a person into which others may not intrude unless they have some legitimate reason.

Many nursing procedures involve this personal territory. Some procedures are of so intimate a nature that normally no other person is permitted to carry them out. For many patients the last time such intimate contact was encountered was through their parents. The very act of washing a patient brings the nurse into such close proximity that some patients feel decidedly uneasy. Procedures involving the sexual areas of the body may present even greater difficulties. Contact (and this is not necessarily physical; exposure to the eyes is a very potent form of contact) in these areas is generally reserved for a specific purpose and for specific people. Nurses, when they have overcome their shyness, can become rather blasé about intimate contact (including exposure of the patient) without fully realizing the emotional impact this may have on the patient.

When two people make physical contact they are both free agents, and at any time may move away and create a safe distance if they so wish. This mutuality is important, for it is something which is absent in the nurse–patient relationship. The patient has been forced, by his condition, to submit to all manner of physical contact; some of which could violate his ideal sphere. He cannot move away, as he may do under different circumstances, but that does not mean that he always welcomes and accepts it. He may endure rather than accept.

One could imagine that these difficulties of contact would arise between people of the opposite sex. Some people reject contact with their own sex even more strongly than contact with the opposite sex which may be one reason why many female nurses prefer to work on male wards. There may be reasons other than physical contact for this preference, but it should not be discounted.

The way patients react to this enforced intimacy will obviously vary with each individual. Reaction may be verbal or nonverbal. Very few would ever say, "Nurse, I don't like what you are doing", that might make them feel silly. It might be difficult, perhaps impossible, for a patient to give a coherent answer as to why he didn't like such intimate contact. Could a male patient say, "because I feel you might hurt me"—or a female patient say to a male nurse, "because you might assault me"? Very few would feel able to verbalize their feelings in this way. If encouraged to do so, they may only be able to say that the contact made them feel uneasy. When there is fairly close contact between nurse and patient, conversation between them tends to be superficial, thus indicating that what is happening is detached, and that the usual meanings associated with such intimacy do not apply.

Not only may there be ambiguity surrounding what is happening and what is being said, but conversation between patients may indicate heightened feelings. The banter which flies around the ward is often a way of releasing tension. The male patient who has just been attended to by a pretty nurse is sure to have his leg pulled. And the "Wait till we see your missus" in reality allows them all to laugh about what, in other circumstances, could be a threat.

Nonverbal reaction is just as significant as words. Every nurse is trained to observe the patient, but with a clinical interpretation in mind. The patient who lies in bed with his legs drawn up may have abdominal pain; the patient who shades his eyes may be sensitive to light, and so on. But there are other nonverbal cues which indicate feelings. The patient who objects to having the bedclothes removed may be saying, "Don't expose me", or the patient who gets as far away as possible from the nurse may be saying, "Don't hurt me". The patient who, while having his pressure areas treated, cannot relax may feel totally unable to tolerate that degree of physical contact. Physiotherapists are often aware that this barrier against physical contact exists and that it interferes with treatment. If physiotherapy is to be effective, the patient has to be helped to relax. In other words, the patient and the person giving treatment must co-operate and co-operation depends on effective communication.

Counselling—part of treatment

Much of what has been said thus far, in this chapter, is by way of laying the foundation for a more detailed discussion of what is actually involved in patient counselling. There are many instances where counselling patients would be the most appropriate and significant part of their treatment. Relatives should be included in any consideration of patient counselling. So often they are left to cope with the anxiety and the trauma, the fears and worries, at times when they most need help. It is possible, by careful, attentive listening, to reduce anxiety in both the patient and his relatives.

Listening is an essential part of counselling but effective listening is more than a passive exercise. It is active and energetic. The patient who telephones the ward, the day before his admission, and asks "Do I have to bring pyjamas?" may want to talk over his fears about the operation. The female patient who constantly wants to telephone her husband "To ask about the children" may, in fact, be terrified that her husband has found another woman. The nurse who is alert and who has learned to read the many signs, is in a good position to do something to alleviate these anxieties.

Helping the patient to cope with his condition may be spread over a considerable period. Most patients will certainly require information, and the amount of information will vary according to each individual. Some would be satisfied with a simple explanation. Others would be satisfied with nothing less than the full facts. If the patient is expected to co-operate in his treatment, he must be involved in every aspect of it, and information is a vital factor in securing involvement and co-operation. There is some information which is basic and essential. Other information may be imparted if the patient asks for it, or needs it to help him understand more fully what is happening or going to happen.

In the past, patients, by and large, were kept very much in the dark about their treatment, almost as if it were a sinister secret. This was possibly in the belief that the majority would not understand, and if they did, such information would increase anxiety, not allay it. There are those who believe that the patient has a basic right to be told exactly what he *needs* to know, and he should be the one to decide how much or how little. This is supported by Barkes (1979), "In essence this should mean that the doctor has a duty to educate his patient so that he can make the decision for himself." When patients ask, and keep on asking, about something connected with their treatment, is it more information they require, or an opportunity to explore some anxiety? That is where active listening comes in, but as Barkes goes on to say, "The patient should be allowed to stay uninformed if he wishes to and not be forced to listen to explanations."

Joseph (see p. 5) duly arrived, and it was obvious to all that he was going to be the life and soul of the ward; very quickly he had everyone amused. Later that evening the staff nurse noticed that he was lying with the sheets over his head. She observed him for a few moments then picked up some papers and went to his bedside and spoke to him. It was several seconds before he emerged. She asked him some detail which was already on the admission form and when he had given the answer she said,

SN: Is everything all right?
J: Yes, thank you staff.
SN: You've gone very quiet, not happy like you were earlier on.
J: You noticed, then?
SN: Yes, are you worried about something?
J: Oh, I expect you'll think it's silly, but I'm not sure what's going

to happen. I mean, I know I'm to have a cartilage taken out but nobody's ever told me what that means.

(The staff nurse explained briefly about the operation, what it would mean and the treatment afterwards.)

SN: You say no one has told you this before? I thought Doctor ... spent some time talking to you earlier today?

J: Yes, he did and now you have told me I do remember him saying much the same thing, but I think I was too nervous to take it in. Tell me, does it really mean that I won't be able to bend my knee again? He did say that didn't he?

SN: You're afraid you will be disabled, is that it?

J: If I can't bend my knee it will stop me playing sport.

SN: You must have misheard the doctor. Your knee should be as good as new after the swelling and pain have gone. You'll have exercises to do, of course, but there's no reason why you should not do as well as Mr Carpenter over there, who has had the same operation. I don't think he's asleep yet, why not ask him. He's due to go home in a few days.

This illustrates how a few minutes listening helped to relieve anxiety. It also shows how information, even when given, is not always accepted because emotions interfere with reception. It also emphasizes that the information may have to be repeated several times before it is received.

The need to understand

In every clinical area different emotional needs may be expressed. It is obvious, when one considers, that the emotional needs of patients in, say, a gynaecology ward are vastly different from those in an orthopaedic ward; and those in terminal care from those in a casualty department. Nurses working in various specialties develop special skills to deal with the multitude of conditions they meet. With each condition the patient needs help in different ways if he is to understand and cope with his condition and the treatment involved.

Understanding and acceptance

One aspect of understanding is what could be called 'understanding by exception'. This means that often instructions are given which tell the reader what to do and what not to do, but do not say what would happen if the instructions are not carried out faithfully. It would not require many additional words. Indeed, too long an explanation could lessen the impact of the message. It has already been indicated that patients often require more than just information presented to them. If their treatment is to be effective, they must accept, emotionally as well as intellectually, what is being said. They also need to be fully aware of what is likely to happen if the instructions are not faithfully carried out. This awareness should come from explicit understanding and not understanding by exception. Joseph was told about his knee operation, but there were reasons why he did not fully understand. His fears got in the way and made him emotionally deaf. Only when the staff nurse repeated the information and dealt with his fear of permanent disability did he remember what the doctor had told him. But, at the same time, the staff nurse did indicate that his full recovery would depend on the way he applied himself to his exercises; this is something Joseph would be likely to hear repeated many times following his operation.

Understanding and adjustment

The patient who is about to have an amputation, however, is in a very different position. For him, there will be a permanent disability with a consequent change in his identity—how he feels about himself. There are many questions to be asked and answered just about the operation and the subsequent treatment, all of which have emotional implications. Many of these practical and psychological issues may involve the relatives as much as the patient. Often an amputation is traumatic and not planned. There is unlikely to be time to explain, to get understanding and acceptance from the patient. The adjustment he must make may be influenced by the way he is helped to cope with the physical and emotional trauma. Though it is true that all members of the team have a part to play in helping to relieve the anxiety, the nurse is the one who has the most sustained contact and this places her in a unique position of being the one to whom he may turn.

There are many excellent books which help the nurse to consider the psychological as well as the physical needs of patients and in an examination, the examiner would certainly look for evidence that the candidate had considered the patient as a whole person and not just as a 'case'. The fact that the psychological needs are written about in textbooks and included in examination papers does not guarantee that those needs are always met. Much of what is read becomes only theoretical knowledge: for it to become more than theoretical knowledge it must be put into practice. A person can learn all about driving a car by reading books but he will find it vastly different when he actually puts his hands on the steering wheel. People can read all there is to be written about nursing, but not until they put into practice what they have read will this become an integral part of their experience.

The same occurs in patient counselling. Nothing succeeds like success; and success comes from practice. There is nothing intrinsically difficult about counselling. It is not a mysterious activity which only super people can do. Much of what nurses do when talking to patients or their relatives could be called counselling, at least within the definition given at the start of this chapter.

Counselling, therefore, may be considered at different levels and each level will require different skill and experience on the part of the nurse. The nurse who says, "Mr Jones, you don't look very happy today; is something worrying you?" and then discovers that he is extremely worried because he is going home next day, but lives 12 miles out in the country, not on a bus route, and cannot afford the money for a taxi, and who makes arrangements for hospital transport, is counselling. She is helping the patient to express anxiety, then helping towards a solution. The nurse who encourages a young patient to talk about the abortion she has just had, with all her guilt and doubts, of how her parents and others reacted and of the young man who promised to marry her then didn't want to know, is counselling. Not only by listening but also by encouraging her to talk about sensitive and painful areas in an atmosphere of acceptance and noncensure. Such incidents may be everyday occurrences, but there are times when, because of the nature of the problem, the nurse would need to counsel at a different level.

Counselling relatives

It has already been suggested that relatives often require as much counselling as patients. It is not always easy, or possible, for the nurse to give time to the relatives when she is so busy attending to the patient. Most nurses would agree that some relatives can be very awkward and demanding. But even the pleasantest persons may become awkward, demanding and irrational when under stress. Relatives of patients are usually under stress, and the severity of the patient's condition may bear no relation to the degree of stress and anxiety the relative feels.

Hospitals may be totally alien to them and they can be fairly awesome places. It was indicated on p. 8 how words may arouse emotions. 'Fever hospital', for one man, always arouses in him a strange mixture of emotions and half-remembered and painful memories of 3 months of early childhood spent in isolation with diphtheria in a fever hospital. Hospital is another world, which may appear strange and frightening. Relatives may have been given only scant information with little explanation. The reason why the patient has been admitted must be considered and all that that could mean to the relationship between the relative and the patient. The relative has to learn a new language in order to communicate with the medical and nursing staff. There is likely to be a great deal of strange-looking equipment which may provoke anxiety. It could be that the only time the relative saw such a machine was on the television, in a programme where the patient had a heart attack and died. The patient's children may have wanted to come, but their mother didn't think that was allowed and she left them at home in tears. It is natural that such a relative's level of anxiety will be raised and she may react in a petulant, demanding and seemingly unreasonable manner, or she may be sullen, resentful and withdrawn. It may be quite true that someone has told her about her husband's condition. The fact that she is now repeating the questions should tell the nurse something, either about her intellectual grasp or about her level of anxiety or a combination of both.

There are some people whose intellectual grasp may make it difficult to explain things to them in terms they can understand. But that is one of the skills of communication—of being able to put things in such a way that the other person does understand. There are others who normally would understand, whose intellectual ability would be adequate to cope with the information, but who experience difficulty in grasping explanations because of heightened emotions at the time. The one may have difficulty expressing herself—it may be something she is not accustomed to doing; the other, who normally may be able to converse quite freely, may still find great difficulty when it comes to talking about her fears and anxieties.

The nurse who encourages relatives to talk does a great service to the relative, of course, but also to the patient. The worry and anxiety experienced by a relative is almost sure to spill over and affect the patient. When this occurs, the patient has a double dose of anxiety. And the reverse is true. If the patient's feelings are inadequately dealt with, they are almost bound to influence the relative. But even if the anxiety of only one of them is dealt with, then the overall level of stress will be lowered and this in turn must have a beneficial effect on the patient's progress.

Who benefits?

Who benefits from the nurse developing counselling skills? First, the patient and/or his relatives; second, the nurse; third, the staff, and last, the organization. How the patient and his relatives may benefit by being able to talk about how they feel, has already been discussed, but there is more to it. What the nurse does is to demonstrate a skill which, hopefully, the patient himself or his relative may be able to exercise, albeit in an elementary way, in the future. The nurse sets an example of how to listen and how to deal with feelings. In the same way as she demonstrates certain clinical techniques, so she demonstrates a particular cluster of skills which we call counselling. There is also a very strong and demonstrable link between counselling and the nursing process.

Counselling and the nursing process

The four stages of the nursing process are similar to the counselling model used in this book. The nurse who said, "Mr Jones, you don't look very happy today, is something worrying you?" is making an assessment and she certainly helped him to plan, by thinking about hospital transport. Then the plan was implemented. Her evaluation would probably be along the lines that Mr Jones looked relieved and was grateful for the solution which he readily accepted. The nursing process demands of the nurse a highly developed ability to relate to people and to assess their physical, psychological and social needs. The nurse, using this method, needs to be a skilled interviewer which is an essential requirement of counselling.

In the assessment stage of the nursing process, a great deal of information is required, for it is here that the relevant details of the patient's nursing and social history emerge. Just how this information is gleaned is important. It is not enough to work through a check list of items to be covered, though it is essential to get all the details. It is possible that this data-gathering will not be achieved at one sitting. What is even more important than the details about occupation, children and family, is the attitude of the patient linked to those details; the quality of the relationships he has with his family, etc. The alert nurse, taking a nursing history, will very quickly pick up cues of sensitive areas. The gap left in dates, the hesitation when speaking of certain persons, the way one child is never mentioned, may all be indications of stress and anxiety which may have a bearing on treatment.

Sandra Osman, a third-year student, while taking a nursing history, noted what she thought was an omission. Mr Link had said he had five children and then went on to give details of their various careers and it was obvious that he was very proud of their achievements but there was one missing. Sandra said, "I think I must have been confused, did you say you had five children? you've told me about four; am I right?" Mr Link was silent for quite a few minutes then said, with tears in his voice, "Yes, Tom, he's in prison, waiting trial for killing someone. It's all dreadful and not something I usually talk about. Do you mind if I tell you about it?" He told Sandra of the pain and hurt, voicing the feelings of the whole family about this tragedy.

While this is not directly concerned with the details of the nursing process, it demonstrates how data collection can uncover needs which are not always apparent. There was nothing that Sandra could actually do; the situation was as it was. By talking about it, however, Mr Link was able to share his grief; more importantly, he had allowed Sandra to get near him emotionally. If he had not been able to share this, it could have become an emotional barrier, but Sandra had been able to establish rapport which permitted this sharing to take place. A person who consciously raises a barrier tends to keep people at a distance, in case they should get behind the barrier and discover what is being kept secret. With such a person, physical treatment and procedures may also present a threat. Treatment may thus be impeded, for with every physical treatment there are likely to be emotional implications which have to be recognized and dealt with if that treatment is to be fully effective.

One aspect of the nursing process is that it depends a great deal on communicating with patients and being able to establish relationships on a different plane to that customary in nursing. Much of what has been discussed in this chapter is about relationships which are influenced, to a great extent, by the level and depth of communication established. The nurse would certainly include in her assessment the quality of the relationships that the patient has been able to establish and with whom. But how is this information obtained? A questionnaire could be devised to supply all this information but this would be but a skeleton. It would not provide the muscle, nerves and blood vessels which are necessary to make a skeleton come to life. A face-to-face talk will provide much more than details. The nurse who herself experiences difficulties with relationships may not find it easy to encourage patients to explore the relationship they have with other people. Her own foundations may not be secure enough to permit her to do this. On the other hand, the nurse who is skilled at establishing relationships and understands what is happening is more likely to perceive indications that the patient's own relationships are suffering from strain and will thus have a more secure foundation from which to act as counsellor.

The needs of relatives

When considering the needs of the patient, the needs of his relatives cannot be ignored, just as one must not overlook the needs arising from the particular clinical condition. One area to which attention should be directed is the patient's age, for at different stages of life, the counselling needs will vary. As the needs of the patient differ, so will the relative's needs be different according to his own age and the age of the patient. The basic need is for understanding and the opportunity to express and explore feelings and fears.

There would be specific differences, for example, between the needs of two mothers, one whose child was suffering from a broken leg and the other whose child was suffering from leukaemia. Similarly, the needs of two elderly male patients—one who has an equally aged wife and no children, the other, a widower with a middle-aged daughter, who lives miles away from her father—again may be very different. Anyone could elicit these facts by means of a questionnaire, but all the dynamics, the hidden meanings, the undertones would be missed. What must constantly be guarded against is assuming that because person A feels the way he does, given an identical set of circumstances, person B will feel and react as A. What that goes hand-in-hand with is a tendency to impose on B the solution which applied to A. It is certainly true that one is able to use the experience gained with A to postulate that B *may* feel and react in a similar way, and to suggest that the solution may also apply. At all times the inference must be tentative.

Take the second example mentioned above. It could be assumed that the daughter would be worried that her father did not have anyone to look after him when he came out of hospital. But, on taking the nursing history, the nurse could very well discover that the old man and his daughter had never enjoyed a workable relationship and that there had been little contact over the years. The nurse may also realize that he is cantankerous and difficult and that any suggestion to send him to his daughter would be resisted by both of them. On talking to the daughter, it may be discovered that although the daughter does feel a sense of guilt, and yes, she is worried, she also realizes that it would be unthinkable for them to live together. So, both father and daughter may need an opportunity to explore how they feel about each other and to be able to look at what such a course would mean to them both. The nurse may not be able to help them explore these feelings at any great depth, yet what she is able to do is often therapeutic. How many times have we heard someone say, "Just talking about it has helped me feel better"?

The patient and his relatives may benefit from counselling, so may the nurse. Just as the patient has general needs and needs specific to his condition, and these are shared (albeit in a different way) by his relatives, so the nurse also has general needs and needs specific to each and every individual patient. Counselling, to stress the point once more, is concerned a great deal with relationships. And in order for the nurse to understand what relationships mean, it is necessary that she understands herself. But she cannot understand herself in isolation. When the nurse forms satisfying relationships, or when she deals constructively with the pain when relationships break down, she understands something more about herself. She has the opportunity to look at what it is about herself that contributes to a satisfying relationship, or contrariwise, what it is that contributes to the breakdown of her relationships.

The needs of the nurse

As nurses operate the nursing process they may discover that many of their own needs are brought to the surface.

Joan, a staff nurse, admitted a young married woman, Sheila, for gynaecological investigation. As they talked, Joan became increasingly anxious as she listened to Sheila, who seemed very unsure of her relationship with her husband. Sheila appeared to be a very negative person with a sharp, critical tongue. Joan was glad when she was called away. Talking this over later, one of the other staff said, "She sounds a bit like you, Joan. You and Terry don't get on well, do you?" Joan became quite annoyed at this remark. Later that week she sought out the occupational-health sister and talked it over with her. To her she could admit that her colleague's remark had been too near the truth for comfort.

Through this one incident Joan achieved a bit more insight into her own reactions, but it is possible that she had more areas to explore. The quest for self-awareness is never fully achieved. If Joan had not met Sheila, it is possible that this insight could have been missed. It is also true that Sheila's needs, just at that moment, could not be met, because of Joan's own anxiety. If Joan had not sought the help of someone else, it is possible that some other patient, in the future, would not feel able to talk about her feelings to Joan. As it was, Joan felt she could be more objective because of her counselling session. Every clinical condition makes specific counselling demands on the nurse, as the next extract shows.

Angela, a midwife, was on duty one night when Sarah was born—the third child of Marion, aged 38. Angela was distressed to observe that Sarah showed every indication of mongolism but felt she could not tell the parents then. She spoke to the doctor next day and he examined Sarah. Marion and Albert were delighted with Sarah receiving so much attention. "You are all so kind and considerate." The doctor asked Angela if she thought she could cope with telling the parents.

Would you stop a moment and think how you would do this? Is there more to this than just 'telling' someone? A person may be told with sensitivity and care, but that is only part of it. Very often the counsellor has to help the other person to frame the questions which need to be asked. There may be a whole gamut of emotions to be explored and worked through—not all at once, naturally. The nurse who uses a counselling approach will make contact with many different emotions. Some of them may cause reverbations within her; some of her own emotional chords may be set in vibration by the emotion of the other person. Every patient or relative, with whom the nurse engages in counselling, offers a potential for further insight and understanding of how she reacts and interacts. And thus, her development as a nurse, and equally important as a person, may be enhanced.

If the patient, his relative and the nurse, may all benefit from counselling, the cumulative gain is that the organization may also benefit. The organization in this instance is the institution which brings patient and nurse together. It may be a hospital, a school, a factory or a patient's home and family. If the outcome of a counselling approach results in a lowering of tension, coupled with increased understanding and insight, and if both patient and nurse benefit, then it is logical to assume that the organization will benefit. If, as a result of counselling, a factory employee feels more able to cope with some domestic crisis, this must surely be beneficial to all concerned. The school nurse who counsels a parent about her child with poor health, contributes to the overall well-being, not only of the family, but of the school. The more that can be done to improve the well-being of individuals should contribute towards healthy and well-balanced organizations which form society.

Nursing, as a profession, must surely benefit if the nurse is recognized as a person who counsels as part of her clinical role. If there is benefit to the individual nurse there will be a cumulative benefit brought about through increased awareness and understanding of how patient needs are related to her own.

Acceptance and rejection

Much of what has been said thus far has been directly concerned with the assessment stage of the nursing process and it has been emphasized that this stage, far from being routine, is in reality complex, because it is concerned with much more than eliciting information. The nursing process implies a much greater involvement in many aspects of the life of the patient. This stresses the importance of acceptance and its close relative, rejection. Elsewhere these two words, as applied to counselling, are discussed, and particularly how possible it is to reject the client because of some aspect of his behaviour (Stewart 1979). The more the nurse becomes involved and the more she gets to know the patient, the more contact she will undoubtedly make with his emotions. A consequence of this increased emotional contact is that the risk of rejection may be increased at the expense of acceptance. The more one knows about another person, the greater the chance there is of something emerging which will conflict with one's own values and principles.

> John, a student psychiatric nurse had been working on his new ward for about a month when he came to see his tutor to ask for a ward change. He was reluctant to discuss the reason why, and hedged round the subject. The tutor got him talking about the type of ward, the staff, workload and so on; none of these things seemed to present any problem. She suggested that if it was none of these, and if, as he said, his personal life was fine, then perhaps the problem lay with the type of patient. Gradually it emerged that there was one patient in

particular who bothered him. The patient, Andrew, who found that he could talk quite easily to John, let it slip (or so John thought) that he was involved in drug pushing. He said, "I found myself hating him." There was no record in Andrew's notes of this fact; John checked. John felt trapped. Should he keep this to himself or report it? His tutor helped him to see that whatever Andrew did was only part of the problem. What John had to do was to come to terms with his feelings of rejection. She pointed out that he did not have to approve of aberrant behaviour in order to accept him. She helped him to see that he could still accept Andrew as a person and at the same time reject his behaviour. He could not approve of his drug pushing; he could reject that, but at the same time he could accept Andrew as a person. She also helped him to explore his feelings of frustration, anger and disappointment at being placed in this position. It would have been easy to change his ward but one questions if that would have been the right solution.

The situation was not resolved in one session but John came through it with a great deal more insight. He was able to pick up the threads of his relationship with Andrew and explained his dilemma (of not wanting to break confidentiality) and not knowing what to do. Andrew respected John's position and took the initiative by telling the doctor of his activities.

This short illustration shows how one nurse dealt with the problem of rejection. The more the nurse moves away from a strict clinical role to include working with relationships, the more possible it is that areas of potential rejection will emerge. While the assessment stage of the nursing process is vital, all the stages are interrelated and it should be thought of as a circular, rather than a linear, process. None of the stages is separate and complete of itself.

When nursing treatment is being planned, due note must be taken of inputs from many sources and it should never be taken for granted that the patient will do what is expected of him. We saw, in the case of Mary and John, on p. 7, how emotional acceptance is necessary if treatment is to be successful.

Mrs J was a stabilized diabetic, aged 70, who worried her son and daughter-in-law because she never went out of the house. The community nurse called one day to discover that Mrs J, although taking her tablets, did not stick to her diet and did not test her urine. She explained to Mrs J why it was important to eat correctly and to regularly test her urine. She said afterwards to one of her colleagues, "I might just as well have talked to myself. I knew she wouldn't do it."

When the nurse got to know Mrs J better, and the old lady was able to talk freely to the nurse, it gradually emerged that she had a physical distaste for handling the urine. She laughed wryly at this, "I've mucked out cows and pigs often enough, and had five kids and all that means, you know, but I just don't like touching that—it's like poison." She was doubtful when the nurse suggested wearing gloves, but agreed to give it a trial. She did, and was delighted to record success. Her diet remained a problem but the nurse felt that with support, Mrs J could cope now that she was testing her urine.

There is nothing very dramatic in this and probably most nurses, at some time, have been faced with the problem patient who has refused to implement his treatment. That is why it is stressed that all four stages of the nursing process are interdependent. In the case of Mrs J, it is doubtful that her distaste of handling urine would have emerged in the assessment stage. Only when implementation of treatment was breaking down did one more part of the assessment picture emerge, but it may not have done so had not the nurse adopted an exploratory, problem-solving approach.

Evaluation is vital

Evaluation, the final stage in the nursing process, puts everything under the spotlight. Then will be revealed success or failure, accuracies and inaccuracies. Attached to these may be praise and, sometimes, unfortunately blame and recriminations. Evaluation is seldom easy; and certainly in counselling it is one area which is often neglected. The more difficult or the less successful the counselling appeared to be, the more likelihood that evaluation will be skimped. In counselling, the client must certainly be involved in the evaluation process and, as has already been indicated, this is or should be, an on-going activity. It is not something left only until the end. If evaluation of the nursing process or of counselling is on-going and if the other person is involved, evaluation will become a dynamic activity, related to the present and not to events of the past.

Evaluation in counselling may prove difficult because the counsellor's own contribution is being examined. Some clients are reluctant to enter into this evaluation; more so if counselling has not been very productive. If things have gone well, if rapport has been established with empathic understanding and if insight has been achieved, positive feelings will be very evident and will no doubt be freely expressed. But what of negative feelings, of disappointment, time wasted, resentment? The client may have difficulty expressing these at any time but if evaluation is left until the end, he may never express them at all. If this happens, he could depart with an overload of negative feelings towards the counsellor and counselling. What of the counsellor's own negative feelings? He may experience the whole range of feelings experienced by the client; intensified possibly by feelings of responsibility and failure. If evaluation is continuous, negative feelings can be explored more readily. It is negative feelings which so often get in the way of effective treatment of the patient. John had negative feelings towards Andrew (p. 22), but when these were explored, balance was restored. Patients must be involved, totally, in all the stages of the nursing process, no less than clients need to be involved in evaluating what takes place in counselling.

Self-knowledge

Discussion, thus far, has centred mainly on the benefits to the patient or his relatives when nurses develop counselling skills. Implicit in this, however, is the benefit to the nurse herself. Alexander Pope said,

> Know thyself, presume not God to scan:
> The proper study of Mankind is Man.

If we are to know ourselves, we must study ourselves in relation to other people. The more we understand them, the more we shall understand ourselves. If nurses are to try to meet the patient's physical, emotional and spiritual, as well as his clinical, needs, they must work towards knowing themselves. If they do not seek self-knowledge, many of the patient's needs will go unmet because they are not recognized. Perhaps needs remain unrecognized when the nurse is unable to get to grips with some part of herself. Self-knowledge is never complete; it can never be absolute. No one can ever say "I have arrived", but "I am arriving". Every new patient, every relative, indeed, every new contact, has the potential for fresh discovery. Every day a person lives, every journey he takes, may open another door to his inner self, if he allows it to happen. He can allow it to happen by not pushing other people away or by keeping them at clinical arm's length.

Everyone has the right to say, "I don't want to know myself or to know how I relate to other people, or what makes me and them tick." Just as the patient has the undeniable right not to know or not to be given information about his condition or the right to keep things to himself if he so wishes, so does the nurse have this right in relation to self-knowledge. Self-knowledge must be sought; it can never be forced by one person onto another.

Summary

This chapter discusses how patients and their relatives can be helped, by counselling, to co-operate fully and with understanding in the treatment regimen. Co-operation does not depend on blind compliance but rather on acceptance and understanding at both intellectual and emotional levels. Decisionmaking, which involves the patient, is linked to the patient's rights to know, to be given information if he so wishes but not to have it forced upon him. The information required by patients, or their relatives, needs to be communicated in such a way that it is understood. The nurse needs to know that understanding has been achieved. In this context, the different levels of communication are examined and how information-giving and receiving are influenced by the content, meaning and emotional overtones. Some aspects of nonverbal communication are touched on, particularly physical contact which features significantly in nursing practice. Listening, an essential charcteristic of counselling, is shown to be a dynamic, active process, rather than being passive.

It was proposed that there are a number of benefits, of developing counselling skills; to the patient—or/and his relatives—and to the nurse herself. Benefits to the staff as a whole, to the organization and, ultimately, to the nursing profession at large, are mentioned but are not covered in depth. Counselling, as an activity, is related to the four stages of the nursing process. It was shown that the depth of skill required when using the nursing process could be enhanced by training in counselling; for the two activities have similarities. If the nurse does not develop understanding and insight related to her own emotions, and how to deal with relationships at more than a superficial level, the nursing process, where implemented, may be ineffective. Counselling may thus be seen to make a positive contribution to patient care.

References

Barkes, P (1979) A Report of the Oncology Society's Annual Conference in Oxford, Nursing Standard, 19 April 1979

Chomsky, N (1968) Language and Mind, Harcourt-Brace Jovanovich

Hall, E T (1959) The Silent Language, Doubleday

Stewart, W (1979) Health Service Counselling, Pitman Medical, p 54

CHAPTER 2

MEETING THE CLIENT

The model introduced

The chapters which follow, introduce the reader to the Wessex model of counselling.* Before going on to 'meet the client'—the first stage of the model—it is necessary to say a few words about why a model is used at all.

---

*The title does not imply that the model was developed by or for any official organization or body which has 'Wessex' in its title. It was so named because the author lives in Wessex.

The model in nursing

It was indicated in the previous chapter that nurses are already familiar with the model of the nursing process. The model of counselling to be presented is offered as one way of systematically looking at the counselling process. A model is a pattern which other people can use, though the use different people put it to may vary. Some models, as in machine tooling, must be copied exactly, with every detail; others may be modified to suit needs and desires, as when using a dress pattern. A counselling model is certainly never intended to be rigidly adhered to; this would be obstructive and would assuredly hinder creativity. The nursing-process model is one which allows for adaptation and creativity, according to the needs of the patient and the particular setting in which it is being used. A model should provide some basic guidelines; but they should be guidelines and not constraints. A model should have a certain inherent logic. Working to a counselling model, however loosely, can help to ensure that one does not start thinking of a solution immediately the problem is presented. Equally, that one does not encourage the person to start planning what to do before he has had adequate opportunity to explore all the ramifications of the problem.

When the nursing process and the Wessex model of counselling are put side-by-side, they look like this:

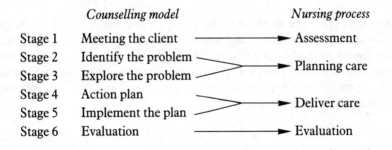

	Counselling model	*Nursing process*
Stage 1	Meeting the client	Assessment
Stage 2	Identify the problem	Planning care
Stage 3	Explore the problem	
Stage 4	Action plan	Deliver care
Stage 5	Implement the plan	
Stage 6	Evaluation	Evaluation

One of the problems of presenting either the nursing process or a counselling model on paper is to convey that it is a dynamic and not a static process, neither does it always follow neatly from start to finish. Another difficulty is to convey that unspoken awareness of when it is time to move on to the next stage. These difficulties are accentuated in counselling, for there is no clearly identifiable point at which to move on. Rather, it is a blending, a merging of what is taking place, that provides a natural impetus for movement forward. This unspoken awareness—so important in counselling, is more easily demonstrated in a teaching group or by listening to interviews.

The nurse–patient relationship

The nurse establishes and maintains her professional relationship with patients on the foundations of trust, respect, understanding and interest. These are precisely the ingredients of the counselling relationship. The respective relationships of nursing and counselling rest more on the personality of the nurse or counsellor than on explicit knowledge. Knowledge and specific expertise are obviously essential for both nurse and counsellor; but expert knowledge must always be tempered with heart-feeling, otherwise the service rendered will be like that described by Keats in,

> Do not all charms fly
> At the mere touch of cold philosophy?
> ....
> Philosophy will clip an angel's wings.

Lamia part 2 line 229

Service, of the kind discussed in this book, if it does not spring from a caring attitude will be mechanical and will lack spontaneity and life. Its recipients are almost certain to sense whence it springs. If nurse or counsellor become mechanical in their service it could be argued that they are not ministering life to the people they serve. Progress and recovery may be seriously retarded by lifeless service.

Meeting the client

The first stage of the model starts with the client. Meeting the client is probably the most vital stage; for it is upon the foundation of this first contact that any hope of productive counselling is built. In these early contacts the nurse and the client set out to establish a relationship in which both feel comfortable and feel that they are able to work together in an area which is causing concern to the client.

Tell me about yourself

What has been said above makes it sound easy and matter-of-fact, but, in reality, the first contact may be difficult. Some clients talk quite readily about themselves and whatever it is that is causing them concern. Indeed, so ready may they be to talk, that listening to them one may wonder, if they find it so easy to talk, why is there a problem? But even in this, caution must be exercised. The glib tongue may portray only surface feelings. The spate of talk may cover up anxiety. Then there is the client who has difficulty expressing himself, and every word seems to be drawn from the depths, with long silences punctuating brief comments. The nurse may be tempted to think, "Oh, do hurry up; say something." If, as in the first instance, the client talks too much, without waiting for some exchange, the nurse may feel like putting a stop to it, and may try, without much success. In both these situations the clients may be reacting like this through nervousness. But why should they feel nervous?

People who counsel are usually warm and caring people, not awesome and frightening; but the clients do not really know this until they arrive. It may have taken a great deal of courage to make contact with the counsellor. Part of this may be due to the fact that until one has become involved in counselling, it is difficult to imagine what it is all about. So, reluctance to make contact may be something to do with fear of the unknown. Part of it may be also to do with fear of the known or partly known.

Tell me how you feel

A person may, for many weeks, suffer from some complaint and yet not seek medical help because he does not realize there is anything wrong, except he knows that he feels below par.

Nancy, at the ripe age of 78, began to feel unwell. "I mustn't complain", she said, "It must be my old body wearing out." Various people came and went and each one of them agreed with her that it probably was 'just old age'. One nurse, to whom Nancy got chatting at a coffee morning, asked a few more questions—pointed ones. She had her suspicions! She made a point of speaking to Nancy's general practitioner, to whom she confided her suspicions. The general practitioner visited Nancy and arranged for her to have some blood samples taken. The results confirmed that Nancy had pernicious anaemia. Within weeks of starting her injections, Nancy said "I've been given a new lease of life".

Nancy had tried many times to say how she felt, but she had not been able to convey her feelings accurately enough. Nancy may very well have concluded that she was imagining things, and if nothing had been detected she may very well have experienced an overwhelming hopeless resignation. It is possible that she had tried on many occasions to give the doctor a precise description of how she felt, but as she was unable to point to an area of her body and say, "I have a pain there", it would be difficult for the doctor to get in touch with her feelings. Had she been able to say, "I have a pain there", or been able to give precise details of when the pain was present ("always before meals, and it is a gnawing pain, and I want to vomit") the doctor would have 'had more to go on. Otherwise it may be difficult to determine the exact nature of the complaint. In such a case the patient, because she is unable to identify clearly what is wrong with her, may be put off going to the doctor, simply because she may not be able to be precise. She may also be afraid that something dreadful will be uncovered.

In much the same way, fears and anxieties impede counselling. Counselling is generally a verbal exchange, and there are some people who find it difficult to accept that 'talking' can bring the degree of relief they are seeking. If counselling were just talking, perhaps their reservations would be justified. But counselling is more than talking. This will be dealt with in greater detail later on.

I am a failure

Possibly one of the biggest hurdles a person seeking counselling has to overcome is the feeling of failure. Many people manage to cope with all the changes and difficulties of life without having deliberately to resort to counselling help. It is possible that such people are fortunate in a number of ways: a particular type of personality, an emotionally well-balanced life, friends who are supportive and who lend listening ears and thus act in a counselling capacity. There are other people who do need help, but that does not mean that they are weaklings. It is more likely that at some stage of their lives something, some experience, or some human contact, was lacking, leaving a gap in which their present problem lodges.

Because most people do manage their own affairs and cope with the stresses of life, those who feel unable to manage, are often overtaken by guilt that they have not been able to 'captain their own ships'. This feeling of guilt, which is often coupled with a sense of failure, may make them even more reluctant to seek counselling help, in just the same way as many people with physical complaint often put off visiting their doctors, saying

"Perhaps it will go away" or "Perhaps I'll overcome it." In some cases this does happen, and their problems disappear; but in many others, just as the physical complaint often becomes chronic for want of treatment, so the individual with emotional difficulties, who could benefit from counselling, often leaves it until the problem or problems has invaded and influenced many aspects of his life.

Counselling—one more hurdle

It is obvious that there are some people for whom counselling is a last resort; a great hurdle to be overcome. Such people are very likely to approach the nurse with a mixture of mistrust and resentment. These feelings are not generated by the nurse; rather, it is that they arise within the individual—for some of the reasons stated above—and they are then projected onto the counselling process and directed at the nurse. These feelings may make the person behave in a number of different ways. He could be sullen, argumentative and touchy or, realizing that such feelings are unreasonable, he may overcompensate by being talkative, effusive and superficially pleasant, giving the impression of being willing to co-operate. On the other hand, he could be tearful and agitated.

There is also the person who feels under pressure to seek counselling. This pressure may be generated by relatives, colleagues, employers or simply by the situation in which the person finds himself. For example, an employer may consider that his employee is showing signs of stress and recommends that he seeks counselling help from the staff counsellor. The employer's intentions and motives may arise from a genuine caring attitude, but the individual may feel that he is being put under pressure to seek help. In much the same way, a stressful situation may drive a person to the counsellor.

Mrs White lived with her husband and four children on a council estate in a big city. Over a period of about a year, the Whites had complained many times to the local authority of damp in their downstairs rooms. Furniture and pictures rapidly grew mould, and wallpaper rotted. To complicate matters, Debbie, the youngest child of 7 years, developed bronchitis, which the doctors attributed to the unhealthy conditions at home. On one of her visits to the school, Mrs White discussed her problem, very briefly, with the school nurse, who was examining Debbie. Recognizing the stress under which Mrs White was labouring, she arranged to see her at the end of the clinic.

While Debbie was taken care of by one of the staff, her mother and the nurse talked around the problem. At the end of the session, Mrs White went away feeling "... a load has been taken off my shoulders". She had received some very positive help from someone who had a listening ear.

The nurse commented afterwards, "Mrs White, at first, was very defensive and kept saying, 'I want to be able to manage this myself', and in the end it transpired that she felt that her pride had been wounded by admitting that she could not cope." It is possible that if Mrs White's wounded pride had not been acknowledged, she may not have been so ready to accept the offered help.

Showing the way

Having taken into account a few of the factors which may influence the reactions of a person who requires counselling, it is now necessary to look at the person acting as counsellor. It was implied in Chapter 1 that much of the outcome of counselling depends on the quality of the relationship which the counsellor and client establish. This relationship—different from most other relationships—is very definitely the product of what both contribute. It is probably true to say, however, that in the first instance it is the counsellor who shows the way, who demonstrates certain skills which permit and encourage the client to contribute what he feels able.

The counselling contract

When the nurse and client have established that they feel able to work together, it is usual to enter into some form of 'contract' or agreement about how they will proceed. This is particularly important when it seems that more than one session is required. Some readers may jib at the word 'contract'; but what it does imply is an undertaking, on both sides, of how the affair is to be conducted. Some writers suggest that a written contract may be beneficial *for some clients*. Some clients may require a piece of paper before the significance and the importance of the undertaking really registers with them. But for the majority, a verbal contract is sufficient.

The client will agree with the nurse the area to be tackled in broad detail.

For example, the client may be aware that his marrige is shaky, but on no account does he want his wife to become involved. One client may acknowledge that he needs counselling to help him accept the forthcoming amputation of his leg; he may also have difficulty coming to terms with his adolescent mentally handicapped son, but he feels unable to discuss this. Another may request help with her financial difficulties, but not yet feel ready to talk about the recent death of her husband.

So, the contract is a setting of boundaries and expectations. Some clients do not want to set such boundaries; for them, counselling needs to be free-ranging. Such trust places a tremendous onus on the nurse who may, unknowingly, tread on uncharted land; the client, because of the emotional disturbance, may resent this. Some boundaries are usually helpful.

Apart from the boundaries to exploration, there are the boundaries of time. How long will each session last? How frequently will the nurse and client meet, and where? In a fee-paying service the fee will be discussed and agreed. There needs to be a tentative agreement reached on how many sessions should be aimed at and how they will be assessed. A part of the contract should be that the nurse discusses with the client that she herself has regular contact with another experienced counsellor, with whom she may discuss specific difficulties currently being experienced with clients. To some people this may seem as if the client's confidence is being betrayed, but this is not so. Supervision—or the 'mentor relationship'—is accepted as being an essential part in developing counselling skills. The question of confidentiality will be dealt with in Chapter 3.

Stage 1 skills

This section introduces four principal skills which operate throughout counselling:

1. Awareness of the uniqueness of the client.
2. Rapport.
3. Empathy.
4. Listening and questioning.

It could be argued that the first three are qualities rather than skills, but it could be counterargued that very few things in life are inherited and that many are acquired and learned. It is perfectly true that within each person lies certain talents which may or may not have been fully developed. But, generally, even the best talent has to be developed. If it can be trained and developed, then one could say that a skill had been acquired. Just so in counselling. There may be some nurses who are endowed with certain attributes which make them suitable counsellors, but it is also possible that these same nurses have acquired these attributes by being exposed to certain influences throughout their lives. The premise of this book is that the majority of nurses could learn the skills of counselling if they have a genuine desire to do so. But, like any other skill, much practise is required; and a willingness to undertake a great deal of scrutiny of one's performance as a counsellor. This constant examination and re-examination inevitably leads to a greater self-awareness, and hand-in-hand with this comes more understanding of people as clients.

The unique client

It may seem unnecessary to state that every client is unique. Just how this uniqueness shows itself needs to be expanded. There are some obvious areas such as work, male/female, status and so on; and we all attach different emphases to all of these, but there are other areas which, at first glance, may not be so obvious.

Personality.   This book is not the place to enter into a lengthy discourse on personality types and how they are reputed to behave; but suffice to say that because everyone has a different personality, it is fairly obvious that there are likely to be some people with whom the nurse will come into contact, as patients or clients, whose personalities would not be compatible with her own. There may be patients and clients with whom she feels she could be friends, but there are others with whom she could not. But counselling is not, in the strict sense of the word, friendship. The nurse, naturally, must be friendly, but when the ingredients of any constructive relationship (and it is possible to have negative and destructive relationships) are considered, it will follow that these form the bases on which friendships are built. The difference between friendship and counselling is in the reason for the contact, rather than in the quality of the relationship.

Most people have a fairly good idea of their own personalities, though they may not always be able to explain what they mean in psychological terms. They will also know the type of people with whom they feel at ease, and those with whom they clash. Knowing how she may react to different people is a great help when the nurse meets a client. If she knows that she finds it difficult to tolerate the type of individual whose personality is hard and calculating, who does not show much feeling, she can be alerted to how she may react if a client presents himself in this way. If the nurse is sincere, she may find it difficult to tolerate clients who appear shallow and insincere. Nurses who can make decisions in their own lives may find it difficult to cope with clients who are indecisive.

One of the essential components of any counselling training is a continuous development of self-awareness. To know oneself, and how one is likely to react to a particular person, is self-awareness and can only improve relationships. But for the nurse, self-awareness is more than just knowing about herself, and how she may react. Self-awareness is not only knowing the negative aspects of oneself; very often people are but dimly aware of their strong points. Self-awareness means accepting ourselves as we are and, if possible, trying to do something about those areas that may act as obstacles in our relationships. When we accept what our self-awareness has revealed, particularly the less desirable aspects of our inner worlds, the things that have possibly caused us so much difficulty are seen in true perspective and some of the sting will be taken from them.

It is true that the nurse may always be critical, but her criticism is likely to become less damaging when it is tempered with insight and understanding. In other words, self-awareness often removes some of the heat from the fires within us which drive us into conflicts, either with other people or with ourselves. Self-awareness does not make us perfect; it does make us more understanding of ourselves and of others.

Character.   An aspect of personality is character—that sum total of a person's qualities that influence the way he behaves towards others. A facet of character is how one person treats other people, influenced by his moral attitude and his ethical values. Of all aspects of character, it is possible that moral attitude is the one that has the greatest potential for conflict between two people. It would be very unlikely that two people would come together in friendship if their moral codes were vastly different. Yet, in counselling this situation may very well arise. That is why it is essential that the nurse develops the ability to suspend her own judgements so that they do not confront the client's, thus creating conflict. A probation officer, working with a man who had been convicted of child-battering, said that had he not been in the position of counsellor, he was conscious that his own moral code would certainly have made him pass judgement on the man. Judgements often produce conflicts.

Beliefs and prejudices.   Another factor of self which the nurse must consider are her own beliefs and their related prejudices. In many ways these relate to the previous paragraph on moral values and codes of ethics. So often, people believe a specific course of action to be right, and the fervour with which they pursue that course may bring them into conflict, open or disguised, with other people; for example, the case of the child-batterer and the probation officer. There are other beliefs (religious ones, for instance) which may create conflict between people, and in any multiethnic society it is very possible that most nurses will have to deal with people whose religious expression is in sharp contrast with their own.

Motivation.   A person's motivation towards significant areas of his life is something else that contributes towards his uniqueness. There is a natural tendency for some people to assume that because they have achieved a certain thing, that everyone else should likewise be able to.

Unless the nurse has taken account of what motivates her, she could mistakenly apply pressure on the client to move along a certain route, propelled by her own motivation and not by his. This may work for a time, but unless the 'will to change' comes from within the client, change, if it does occur, is likely to be short-lived.

Something very akin to motivation is enthusiasm. The nurse who is enthusiastic by nature may find it difficult to understand the client who appears to have little enthusiasm for anything, especially in trying to work towards solving his problem. Enthusiasm is contagious. In counselling, it can be quickly 'caught' by the client, who is then carried along on the wave of the counsellor's enthusiasm. If this sounds dismal, there is a more positive side. The nurse's enthusiasm, carefully controlled, may kindle or rekindle the spark of enthusiasm in the client. When this happens, the client then develops his own brand of enthusiasm which he will channel in his own way and for his own ends, not for the benefit of anyone else.

Experience.   The last area to be covered in this consideration of the uniqueness of the client is the vital area of his life experience. It is extraordinary, but true, that two children of the same parents may both emerge from that home giving the impression of having experienced two significantly different up-bringings. If this can apply to siblings, how much more may it apply to those who are not related? Two people can look out of the same window and see two dissimilar worlds. Two student nurses can listen to the same lecture and hear quite different explanations of how a certain organ of the body functions. How we perceive the world around highlights our uniqueness. In the same way, what has occupied the waking hours of people exerts different influences. There are those who would argue that not only are waking hours important, but that what goes on in the mind during sleep, exerts a powerful influence when the person is awake. The very nature of a person's daily occupation is a major factor in creating him as he is. A person's thoughts, private to himself, are also a potent factor in this.

Most people slot neatly into occupational pigeon-holes, and are given—or don of their own free will—a set of expectations in keeping with a specific occupation: the 'angelic' nurse, the 'burly' policeman, the 'school-marm'. Having donned this cluster of expectations, most people find that this role takes over to a degree, and it is often difficult for people to break out of their roles. It is also difficult for other people to see the person behind the role. When considering a client, it is essential to look beneath his role, to discover what makes him unique. Many people take refuge in their roles by saying something like, "Oh, I'm only a ..." or "You can't expect me to do that, I am not ..."

There are also those who use their roles to gain, or try to gain, advantage over other people. Most nurses will have experienced being lorded over by a senior nurse, using her position to gain some advantage. There are those who never allow themselves to approach other people emotionally or to be approached; the role is a barrier. When it is realized that many people need something behind which to hide their true selves, counselling will become easier, particularly if whatever they are hiding behind is not harshly or rashly torn away. Removal of a person's psychological defences is not the aim of counselling. Removing defences may leave that person so vulnerable to further internal and external pressures that the resulting state could be far worse than the original. If the nurse can assist the client to stand with her and view the defences from the outside, if the client can get the nurse to stand with him and view the defences from the inside, and if as a result of these fresh perspectives, insights develop which allow the client to function more effectively, counselling will have been productive.

In considering the 'unique client' (and the 'unique counsellor') some important areas have been touched on. There are, no doubt, other important areas that could have been selected, but the discussion may have generated some thoughts and thrown some new light on some familiar topics.

Rapport

The second skill is rapport. This word is used a great deal in any discussion on relationships. It would appear to derive from the special relationship that exists between hypnotist and subject. But in a more general sense it is a "relationship based on a high degree of community of thought, interest and sentiment ..." (Drever 1969). The Webster's 'New World Thesaurus' gives as synonyms for rapport: harmony, compatibility and affinity. The discussion will now concentrate on these three words.

Harmony. Most people would agree that for a relationship between two people to be satisfying, harmony, compatibility and affinity must be present. If this is so for all relationships, then if counselling is a relationship it pertains to that also. It must not be assumed, when speaking of harmony in this context, that absolute harmony is suggested. This would be impossible to achieve. An analogy may be drawn from nature. The relationship of plant life to the rest of the universe is held in delicate balance. At some time in this process of keeping the atmosphere at a fairly constant level of essential gases, absolute balance may be achieved; if it is, it is transitory. The moment perfect balance is achieved, something happens to disturb the balance and the process of rebalancing starts all over. For most of the time, nature is in a state of 'relative harmony'. This analogy fits human relationships very well. In counselling, although harmony is an essential component in rapport, and while it may be achieved, it is likely to undergo fairly rapid and frequent changes, as elements from first one person, then another, come to disturb the balance. Just as nature exerts a continuous pressure to achieve and maintain harmony, so do nurse and client in the counselling relationship. Achieving and maintaining this harmony is a combination of conscious and unconscious elements; but it must be stressed that it does not happen by chance. It is a very active process which must be worked at.

Built into this process of balance and harmony is the idea that there is "no growth without conflict". If nothing ever disturbed the balance in nature, it is very possible that instead of harmony, stagnation would result. Just so in relationships. There are some relationships that survive with only minimal conflict to disturb the balance; in others, the periods of balance are very much shorter, disturbed by conflict of great moment. Provided that there are periods of relative harmony, allowing regrowth to take place, the relationship will probably survive. If, however, the periods of conflict are so disturbing and so frequent that little or no harmony exists, such a relationship will be unharmonious and will stand little chance of surviving, for the one reason, that no space exists to permit regrowth to take place.

What has been said applies also to the counselling relationship. Its very nature implies that two people are brought together because one of them (the client) is seeking help from another person (the counsellor). Attention was drawn earlier to some areas within the client which may produce conflict in the initial stages of the counselling relationship. When rapport has been established, harmony may be disturbed from time to time. As a result of encouraging the client to examine some aspect of his life, conflict may be produced within him which may then disturb the rapport between him and the nurse. But, such conflict is often essential if the client is to make progress. If the degree of conflict is too great, and harmony cannot be restored, counselling may break down.

> Sally had been coming to see Elizabeth for help in coming to terms with not being able to have children. During the course of counsell-ing, Elizabeth elicited the fact that Sally was holding back a great deal of anger. It was obvious, by the way Sally responded, that such exploration was creating conflict within her with which she could not cope, nor could she express her feelings openly. She missed her next appointment, then rang to say that she thought that, for the time being, she had gone as far as she could.

The sensitive nurse will often be aware that the client is experiencing conflict and may be able to take steps to reduce it, by allowing adequate opportunity for expression of feelings, some of which may be directed towards her. But, as was seen with Sally, some clients may still withdraw from counselling. Negative feelings from the client may very well generate conflict within the nurse; such conflict then has the possibility of fresh growth for her. Out of this conflict, harmony can once more be re-established.

Compatibility.   It is difficult to identify the components in two people that make them compatible or incompatible. Possibly it is as much to do with what cannot be identified as with what can. And it is often easier to state reasons why two people do not get on as it is to state why they do. Compatibility ties up with harmony, in as much as if conflict is severe and lasting, without sufficient periods of harmony in which feelings can settle, balance may not be easily restored.

In a nontherapeutic relationship there are several factors which may determine compatibility: personality, looks, intelligence, emotional stability, understanding, kindness and tenderness are some of them. Most people do not consciously work out what it is that makes them compatible with other people. Most of us are quite satisfied to enjoy the company of people with whom we feel comfortable and to avoid the others, but in a therapeutic relationship a different set of rules operate. It is true that the client could search around to find someone with whom he feels instantly compatible. Generally speaking, clients have very limited choice of people who are available; and certainly the opportunity for every client to 'shop around' to find someone with whom he feels instantly comfortable would be unrealistic. This then places the onus fairly and squarely on the shoulders of all who would counsel, to make themselves *as compatible as possible* with as wide a range of people as possible. If this sounds a formidable task, it is, but not a superhuman one. The nurse who reaches out to other people, from a foundation of trust, interest, respect and understanding, is doing everything possible to ensure that the person coming for counsel is able to make contact with a great deal that is positive.

Competition and co-operation.   It was indicated earlier that many things could get in the way to hinder positive contact; one of these is the element of competition. Western societies are intensely competitive and this is obvious throughout all sections from a very early age. This statement will be easily confirmed by studying a group of children playing at school; how they will strive for mastery over other children. It could be argued that this is man's natural tendency, and it could quite well be, but it could also be argued that it is man's natural instinct to kill. He is encouraged in one activity and positively discouraged in the other. It is also possible that competition is a relatively harmless channelling of this primitive drive. At the same time as competition is encouraged, at school, in sports, at work and in many other areas of life, attempts are made to foster co-operation. Undue competition at work may be quite a significant factor in producing intolerable levels of stress in certain individuals.

In a sense, team games fall into a mixed category: co-operation between players is essential, but with a highly motivated competition as the goal. True co-operation (e.g. in a choir or an orchestra, or the building of a house by a team of craftsmen) requires a very different attitude. Perhaps the reason for this is that competition has more excitement, more immediate thrill to it than co-operation; for example, the thrill of the downhill ski competition is immediately appealing, possibly because of the high level of adrenalin produced.

Whatever the outcome, physiological or psychological, the question that must be asked is: Can highly competitive people move easily into an essentially co-operative role? Nursing, by virtue of its structure, is a competitive occupation. At first glance this may not seem to be so, but a closer examination may very well reveal the truth of this. The system of grades and marks, passes and credits, 'ordinary' and 'honours' certificates, and ward reports are examples of how (possibly and unintentionally) the spirit of competition is fostered. Yet, at the same time, the nurse must learn to co-operate with other care-giving staff and with patients. If she does not learn to do this, the patient's needs will not be fully met. This spirit of competition, harmless on the playing-field, may spell disaster in relationships, where, instead of fighting to gain possession of a ball or to score a goal, each person is constantly trying to dominate the other, to gain possession of an emotional ball. Such a couple were Andrew and his young wife.

Both Andrew and Margaret were 21 when they married, after a whirlwind romance. At the time they married, both were taking driving lessons. Margaret was always very critical of Andrew's driving; passing such comments as "You've crashed the gears again", "You slid back on that hill", "You didn't indicate early enough". Andrew tolerated this with good humour, saying, "Well, let's wait till the test." Margaret took her test before Andrew and was bitterly disappointed to fail. Her disappointment turned into anger when a week later Andrew passed. So great was her competitive spirit that even although there was no outright competition, she perceived this activity in this light. She always had to be the winner. Their marriage did not last. This was not the only area of incompatibility, but her competitive spirit, coupled with Andrew's almost total lack of it, was a significant feature in the breakdown.

Nurses who engage in counselling have to co-operate with clients and not compete with them. The nurse who enters into a spirit of competition with the client is sure to end up in conflict with him. It is possible that the seeds of competition lie deeply buried in some emotion or experience that is reawakened by contact with a particular client. On the other hand, if the nurse is someone who always wants to win, always wants to score, always wants to get on top, then co-operating with the client may prove difficult. A client who is prepared to co-operate may very well be swamped by a competitive nurse and be persuaded to make choices that have mental rather than emotional assent. A highly competitive client may try very hard to engage the nurse in a competition, rather than in exploring his problem. If the nurse does not 'play the game', conflict may be generated within the client. This could very well be the spark to kindle the desire to change.

Affinity.   The last of the three components of rapport, affinity, is to do with the quality of the relationship. Analogies may be drawn from chemistry and physics. Two specific elements are attracted to each other to form a compound. It is difficult for a layman to explain in simple terms just exactly why, for instance, two parts of hydrogen and one part of oxygen form water. There is something inherent in the atoms of the two elements that permits this transformation to take place, if the conditions are right. In a similar way, a magnet and iron are attracted to each other. Two people who fall in love and are attracted to each other are said to have an affinity. In law, the term 'affinity' has a precise meaning as distinct from 'consanguinity': the former is the relationship between married people; the latter is the relationship between blood relations.

Counselling is not necessarily built upon attraction between client and nurse, or indeed upon liking each other, in the way that one would be attracted to or would like a potential friend. But at the same time friendliness and some degree of liking are essential. What is more significant, just as in friendship or marriage, is the unique bond that is established between nurse and client.

Several times in the foregoing discussion, reference has been made to the counselling relationship; the bond is part of that relationship. Client and nurse have come together for a specific purpose, and unlike the bonds that hold other relationships together, this one has in its make-up the inevitability of coming to an end. Nurses are conscious of this with patients. Here the relationship can be fairly intimate and at times intense, yet both know that sooner or later the relationship will end. The more one invests in a relationship, the stronger the bond grows and the breaking of it may bring pain. But to compensate, both client and nurse take with them something of the investment of the other person to enrich their respective experiences. As water can be reduced to its component elements, so when the time comes, the counselling bond is dissolved. Counsellor and client separate to go their own ways.

Wave-lengths. To sum up this discussion on rapport it would be helpful to draw one final analogy. Basically it could be said that rapport is established when two people are on the same wave-length. One can imagine two people as radios, each one transmitting and receiving. If person A is transmitting on short wave, unless person B is also tuned to short wave, reception is impossible. Added to this, the tuning mechanism must be finely tuned if the signal is to be picked up. The signal may be deflected and distorted by numerous influences and obstacles, for example, atmospherics and concrete buildings. There are many obstacles to people establishing rapport; many things interfere with the signals. The radio operator who hears a faint, "I can't hear you" may be able to send a stronger signal; the receiver may be able to do some fine tuning and thus receive a clearer message.

If the nurse feels that rapport is not being established, a remark such as "We don't seem to be getting on the same wave-length" may be sufficient to allow both her and the client to stop and examine why. In saying this, however, she should avoid giving the impression that the lack of rapport is the client's fault. Rapport is two-way.

Empathy

The third essential skill is empathy. One of the definitions is "The capacity for participating in or a vicarious experiencing of another's feelings, volitions (actions) or ideas."* From this definition, it emerges that empathy is a capacity, a power of mind, to relate to another person's feelings, actions or ideas. In order to achieve this, one has to develop "... an ability to walk around in the world of the other person"†; to see the world through the spectacles of the other person; to feel how his shoes fit. It would be presumptuous to suggest that any one person could walk totally in the world of another person, to see the world precisely as that other person sees it, or to feel acutely where the shoes pinch. Nevertheless, if the nurse is able to step into the client's world, even for a brief spell, and walk with him for a little way, empathy has been achieved, however transitory an experience it may have been. It was earlier suggested that harmony was never absolute; neither is empathy. No one may say "I have complete empathy" or "I have achieved empathy" any more than a person may say, "I have complete self-awareness." It is a matter of degree, and the degree of empathy present

---

*Webster's 'Third New International Dictionary'. (Actions)—author's parenthesis.
†B.B.C. 'Introduction to Counselling'.

is very much dependent on the particular relationship. Just as harmony is constantly changing—from balance to imbalance—so does empathy in relationships constantly change, depending on the interaction at the moment. It would be unrealistic to think that for a whole session the nurse was in empathy with the client. One of the ways to detect empathy is the ease of movement between counsellor and client. If discussion, which has been at a feeling level, suddenly switches to become an intellectual discussion, empathy has probably wavered. This does not mean that the fault lies with the nurse; it is possible that the client has put a block in the way of further exploration. This will be dealt with at length in Chapter 4. Suffice it to say that the perceptive nurse will take note of this altered empathy—a temporary imbalance—and then seek to re-establish it by opening another channel. Sometimes it is the counsellor who breaks the empathy by treading indelicately on the client's feelings, by not listening or by trying to push the client. Empathy is a tenuous experience.

Stewart (1977) has drawn attention to a distinction between empathy and sympathy. Certainly any counsellor needs to be sympathetic, but clients, if they are to receive constructive help, do not need sympathy. They may look for and expect it, but it may not be what they *need*. Feelings may be running high when the client presents himself and while the nurse endeavours to make contact with these feelings, she must not become swamped by or immersed in them. Sympathy has a tendency to overidentify with feelings, in much the same way as, for example, the strings on a violin will vibrate in sympathy when an identical note is being played on another violin. If the nurse and client are too much in sympathy the point may be reached when the nurse runs the risk of losing her ability to be objective. Thus, sympathy is a subjective relationship, while empathy is a relationship in which the individual has the ability to be objectively understanding. Sympathy means feeling 'for', empathy means feeling 'with' the individual.

This ability to 'feel with' another person does not necessarily rely on having passed through an identical experience. Indeed, it could be argued that this might·prove a hindrance, particularly if such an experience were recent and still causing pain.

Peter Treadmill,* when talking with his counsellor, about his conflict over his mentally handicapped daughter, had difficulty appreciating other people's feelings. Sally used his childhood experience of losing a

---

*See 'A Family Problem at Work', Occupational Health, 12/12/81–1/1/82.

loved dog, to point to the similarity between his feelings then and his present feelings.

Anyone who has experienced deep feelings about anything is usually able to empathize without too much difficulty. Egan (1975) presents some very useful exercises that will increase one's ability to achieve accurate empathy.

The ability to establish and maintain empathy with clients over the whole spectrum of counselling depends, to a great extent, on innate qualities of personality, strengthened by training. Part of this (which may be natural) is the ability to pick up and interpret accurately what is going on within the other person. Some people do seem to have a knack for this; for others, it is acquired, like any other skill, by patient practice. This 'picking up' is known as 'feedback' and is a continuous process between counsellor and client and back again. Sometimes the feedback is verbal; at other times it is nonverbal. Accurate observation of feedback from the client is essential, as one element in empathy. In the next section listening and questioning will be covered in depth, both of which can make or mar both rapport and empathy.

Listening and questioning

Some people mistakenly think that all a counsellor has to do is listen. Although listening is essential, it is not a passive but an active process, involving all the senses and not only the ears. In any communication between people, four factors have to be considered.

1. Use all senses. Listening demands an attitude of readiness and openness, and an expectation to hear something. There is a subtle distinction between listening and hearing. Many people listen, but do not always hear. However intently a deaf person listens, he will not hear. A hard-of-hearing person has to listen much more intently than a hearing person. Both the totally deaf and the hard-of-hearing may lip read and so 'hear with the lips'; sign language may also be used.

2. Language. The analogy of 'hearing with the lips' holds good in counselling, where not only speech is used but all manner of nonverbal communication. It is worth pointing out at this stage that speech arises from the conscious mind but nonverbal language is, to a large extent, from the unconscious. Thus, in communication, two levels are in operation. In counselling, both counsellor and client may find themselves responding to each other's nonverbal communication and not to the verbal. If what is being communicated nonverbally matches the verbal, the messages are said to be congruent. However, if they are incongruous, conflict will be produced in the receiver. The responses he makes is then likely to be to the nonverbal and not to the verbal. If this conflict between the two elements of communication is not resolved, counselling will surely break down. Thus it behoves all who engage in any form of counselling to be aware of how their inner worlds—those secret parts, consciously secret, or unconsciously hidden—influence relationships. The nurse who is aware that she is responding in a certain way towards a particular client, and this is getting in the way of a positive relationship, would be well advised to pay strict attention to her own nonverbal communication as well as to that of the client. It is possible, by studying the way she is reacting, to bring into the conscious mind what hitherto has been only unconscious. It is in this area that all counsellors are likely to need the assistance of a more experienced counsellor.

3. Understand and be understood.   It may seem unnecessary to state how essential it is when communicating that each person understands what the other is saying. This may sound easy and elementary, but it so often happens that misunderstanding occurs because one or the other has not made himself understood. Thus it is frequently necessary to wait for feedback, to make certain that there is understanding. There are many ocasions when a speaker has assumed that what he has said has been received and understood, simply because the hearer has not acknowledged his lack of understanding. It may not always be easy for people to say, "I do not understand". The fact that one person does not fully understand another is often due to unclear thinking on the part of the speaker, rather than some lack in the hearer. Very often, when a person is speaking, he may never have actually put together in quite that way the words he is now speaking. What starts off as a good idea may become distorted in the process between thinking and speaking. Talking 'on one's feet' does not come easily or naturally to all people.

4. Meaning.   People who come for counselling often feel themselves to be in a jumble because their emotions are jumbled. The person who is incensed with anger may be incoherent. A person distressed with grief may not be able to find any words at all. Strong emotions distort the thinking process. The nurse may have to help any client to express himself. Generally speaking, clients are experiencing some disturbance in their emotions. Part of the skill is to get the client to talk and then to encourage him to continue talking, not necessarily in a nonstop flow, but talk interspersed with listening and thinking. This is achieved by making comments, passing observations and asking questions. Part of the skill is being able to read between the lines; hearing the unspoken meaning of the words.

Four golden rules.   There are some golden rules about the way questions are asked.

1. *Open questions.*   Encourge the client to express what he is thinking and feeling.
EXAMPLE. "Tell me, Mr Andrews, how do you get on with your work-mates?"

2. *Closed questions.*   Useful for getting information and facts.
EXAMPLE. "What is your age, Mr Andrews?" "How many children do you have?"

3. *Leading questions.*   Where the action suggested by the counsellor is contained in the question.
EXAMPLE. "If you were convinced that taking this course of action was morally wrong, you wouldn't take it, would you?"

4. *Avoid making statements that sound like questions.*
EXAMPLE. "You quarrel with your wife, don't you?"

Asking questions also assists in clarifying something that is not quite clear. "I don't understand. Do you mean ...?" will usually help the client by letting him see that the nurse is still with him.

Questions normally should be based on material already provided by the client, rather than based on the counsellor's curiosity. Facts may be necessary, but the nurse, unlike taking a nursing history, when counselling, does not require every minute detail in order to arrive at an assessment. Facts may be duly noted, but not to the extent that they obstruct talking. On the other hand, making a few notes may be an effective way of slowing down an excessively talkative client.

Note taking

This would seem a timely place to say something on taking notes. In certain situations, some notes are essential, if only to keep the key issues before one's eyes. Before starting a session, the nurse who says something like, "What do you feel about me taking some notes?" will rarely meet with a refusal. Such notes need only be single words, enough to act as refreshers later in the session. Single words or short sentences can usually be written without taking one's eyes off the client for too long. Referring to the notes from time to time may give the client confidence that what has been noted is there to be used. A few notes taken in this way provide a useful framework if writing up the interview. It is good practice, if one has the time, to write up a complete interview, as detailed as possible. This may sound a daunting prospect, trying to remember who said what and in what order. This is where the notes are a boon. A single word may be enough to recall the order of discussion and the content. The strict discipline of verbatim recording helps to sharpen observations and recall.

Questions should never intrude into the counselling process. They should always be a natural part of what is going on, and the client should always be able to understand the relevance of the question at the time it is asked. There is a time to ask a question and a time not to. A question may occur to the nurse, but a convenient place to ask it may not present itself. If it is introduced later it may have the effect of stopping the flow; almost like trying to turn the clock back. Introducing it may cause the client to stop, especially if he cannot see its relevance. Sometimes it is necessary to go back to a previous stage in the session. "Earlier on you were telling me about ... I wonder if it would be helpful to pick up that thread again", gives a clear indication that the nurse is still interested and still helping to explore the problem. This theme will be picked up again in a later chapter, but it is by the nurse's use of the skills outlined in this chapter and the way she communicates, that she is able to lead the client gently, but with assurance, into identifyng the problem.

References

Drever, J (1969) A Dictionary of Psychology, Penguin, Reference Books R5
Egan, G (1975) The Skilled Helper and Exercises in Helping Skills, Brooks-Cole
Stewart, W (1977) Health Service Counselling, Pitman Medical, p 41

CHAPTER 3

IDENTIFY THE PROBLEM

The process

Several times attention has been directed towards the similarity between the nursing-process model and the counselling model being used in this book. The nurse who engages in counselling will realize that certain of the skills she uses in the nursing process are extended and deepened when counselling. The two elements of rapport and empathy, most certainly used in nursing, are used in counselling in a different way and for a different purpose. The nurse who has pulled out all the stops to make the client feel accepted and free to express himself will have gone a great way along the road towards effective counselling.

When using the nursing process, the actual condition of the patient may have been identified before admission, and putting a diagnostic label on a patient does not necessarily mean that there are no problems for him to work through. This is where a counselling approach can help. There may be undisclosed problems which may seriously affect treatment and recovery from illness (see p. 17). In this second stage of counselling, the nurse helps the client to identify which specific problem, or part of the problem, could be tackled. During the first stage, the nurse may have helped the client to arrive at a fairly accurate assessment of the situation and she may feel that it would be useful and helpful for the client to tackle the problem along a certain line. But when the client is asked, "What do *you* feel is the most pressing problem you would like to tackle first?", the answer may be quite different from the nurse's idea. That is why it is always wise to let the client choose which area to concentrate attention. This might be an appropriate place to refer back to the discussion on the contract (p. 34). There the client's choice acts as a boundary; now it is a definite though indistinct pathway forward.

The emotional jungle

Some clients may not be able to identify what their problem is. They may be in too vast an emotional jungle. What they need is for the nurse to tread the way with them, cutting aside some of the tangled undergrowth to let in some light. Just listening to what the client says may be enough; and from this, certain possible avenues may emerge. Because the client is uncertain and possibly confused, any suggestion of what the problem is should be offered tentatively and not with any certainty. Phrases such as, "It would seem as if ...", "Could it be that ...?" "This is what it looks like to me ... is that how you feel?" may help him to clarify his thoughts and feelings. Put in this way, he has the opportunity to reject what he is hearing if it does not seem quite right. He might not find it quite so easy to reject openly a statement such as "Your problem is that ...", "Now I've heard you, this is what I think should be done."

Part of the skill in identifying the problem is that very often the client introduces one subject, or part of the problem, in order to lead onto something more important. He does this possibly to 'test the water'—"Will she listen?" "Will she be understanding?" "Will she reject me if I tell her the 'whole' truth?" There are many reasons why people do this. Perhaps they do not want to shock the listener; perhaps they feel the need to be drawn out, to show that the person really understands and is listening; perhaps it is an effort on their part to establish rapport and empathy. But whatever the reason, it is a wise listener who asks a mental question, "Is this all, or is there more to follow?" Too rapid an assessment may create a false premise on which to base counselling; only part of the problem may be solved, or none of it.

Ownership

"It's all her fault", said Mr Taciturn, as he faced the counsellor. "She leads me a dog's life. I can't think why. I've done nothing to upset her." As the counsellor listened, she was thinking, "If he talks like that about her to me, what's he like at home? How does he talk to her in front of the children?" To him she said, "You say you have no idea why she is like she is?" "None at all. If the marriage breaks up it's all her fault. I can't reason with her. She's the one who should be here, not me."

Mr Taciturn had difficulty owning up to the problem; owning up to the possibility that perhaps he had some part to play in the difficult marriage.

Many people, when under stress because their emotions are in turmoil cannot see that they have contributed to the problem: they try to push it away, onto someone else.

> Elsie Fairweather, a student nurse in her second year of training, was dismissed for unsatisfactory conduct. Her sickness record was appalling, made up mainly of single days. Her ward reports always reflected that she was absent a great deal without having made contact with the sister. Her excuses were: "The alarm clock broke", "The bus went without me", "I overslept", "My days off were mixed up", and so on. It was never her fault. Misadventure was always thrust upon her by some malevolent superbeing who had a grudge against her. The problem was not her's, or so she thought.

In both these instances, the problem was being pushed aside. Mr Taciturn needed help to realize that his attitude towards his wife and children was a very powerful factor in the strained relationship. Miss Fairweather was never able to accept that her attitude towards life contributed to her downfall. Unless both of them—and all clients—accept the problem as their's, counselling will be a sterile waste of time. Acceptance of the problem 'as mine', just as the alcoholic must reach this stage before he can start to climb out of the pit into which he has dropped, is a vital stage to be reached before effective counselling can really start.

Using other people

Having helped the client identify the problem, it may sometimes seem more appropriate for someone other than the nurse to counsel that person. No counsellor can possibly expect to work with all people who require counselling. Some clients require very specialized help. Sometimes, and many counsellors will admit this, it just seems impossible to get on the same wave-length as the client. In that instance it would be best for all concerned if another counsellor were found.

> Mrs Swift, employed as a ward clerk, suddenly became moody and irritable with everyone at work. Mr Henwood, the charge nurse, became concerned, when on several occasions he found her crying.
>
> **Mr H:**   Mrs Swift, you don't seem happy recently. I'm concerned. Is there anything we can do? Do you want to talk about it?
> **Mrs S:**   You're not satisfied with my work?
> **Mr H:**   I'm sorry. I didn't mean to give that impression. But you used to be so cheerful …
> **Mrs S:**   Now I'm an old misery, is that what you're saying?
> **Mr H:**   (smiling) You know that's not true, but you're not happy, are you? Is it to do with the ward?
> **Mrs S:**   (after a long pause, during which she fished for a tissue to wipe her eyes) Oh, I've just got to tell someone. It's John, my husband, he's gone off with another woman and he wants a divorce.

Mr Henwood spent a great deal of time with Mrs Swift and realized that she needed help beyond that which he was able to give. She agreed to see the hospital social worker who worked with her over a number of months. There were many things Mrs Swift had to understand about her problems;

many unpalatable factors with which she had to cope. Her major problem—splitting up of the marriage—would not go away, it could not be resolved, but she was helped to cope with it and to make a new life for herself. In this instance, because the problem involved many elements, some of them quite complex, it was more appropriate that she worked with a professionally trained person. But, and this is an important point, the process was started by an observant and caring member of staff. Having admitted that she was having difficulties, it was then easier for Mrs Swift to accept working with the social worker. There were other people outside of the working environment to whom she could have been referred, but it was useful to have a skilled counsellor 'on tap'.

This is an example of how a personal problem was dealt with at work. If it had not been dealt with, it is possible that it would have interfered with the way Mrs Swift performed her task. A slightly different position is where there is clear evidence that performance is not up to standard. In such an instance, the nurse manager would have a definite and clear duty to the organization to attempt to help the other person to find ways to improve.

Pearl, a West Indian nurse in her first year of training, always had good ward reports; above average in most points except in the vital area of punctuality. This always pulled her down. The matron (in the days before Salmon) had almost decided that Pearl should not continue training but decided to give her one more chance on Sister Kennedy's ward. Pearl's reputation had preceded her, but Sister Kennedy wanted to be fair and promised Pearl that she would be judged on how she performed while on her ward. Very quickly it became clear that Pearl did not have much idea of punctuality. To arrive on duty within 10 minutes of the others was considered difficult enough but she found the greatest difficulty sticking to any timetable of ward routine, which at times made her unsafe and caused irritation to the other nursing staff.

Sister Kennedy, after a few days observation, took Pearl to one side and put the facts squarely before her and encouraged her to talk about herself. As she talked, especially about her life in the West Indies, Sister Kennedy realized that time had little meaning in the way Pearl had been brought up, and that what they were up against was not wilful disobedience but a very strong familial or cultural influence. She also realized that Pearl, although she wore a watch, hardly every used it, other than to check patients' observations. Another point that became obvious (and she wondered not only why she had been blind to it but everyone else before her) was that Pearl, though she was more often late on duty than on time, never seemed anxious to go off duty either. The more she thought about this, the more she realized that this was another indication of Pearl's timelessness.

Sister Kennedy and Pearl, who was very anxious to conform, knew that it would not be easy to overcome this deeply ingrained casual attitude towards time and time-keeping. Sister Kennedy spoke to one of the other students who lived in the same residence as Pearl, and the three of them worked out a strategy whereby Pearl would be called for in good time to get on duty. The trained staff, for their part, were asked to co-operate by keeping a strict 'punctual/late' time-table and were asked to ensure that Pearl left the ward on time. Sister Kennedy felt that this—leaving the ward punctually—was as important as arriving on time. In addition, a trained member of staff was responsible for checking Pearl's adherence to schedules.

At the end of her allotted time on that ward, Pearl's time-keeping had improved significantly, though everyone agreed that she still had a long way to go. A ploy used on the ward (the patients also entered into the game, much to Pearl's amusement) was that throughout the day, one or another would call out, "Pearl, what's the time?" Because it developed into something of a joke (though it was not conceived of in this way) Pearl was able to cope with it much better, because it matched her sunny, carefree personality. Sister Kennedy was highly gratified, when the time came for Pearl to move to another ward, that her regimen was adopted in principle by the new staff and the improvement, started on her ward, continued in the new.

Some people would question whether this is counselling and perhaps, strictly speaking, it is not. But what it does demonstrate is a caring attitude on the part of Sister Kennedy and, like ripples on water, her influence spread to many other people who all had a part to play in Pearl's professional development.

It has already been indicated that in counselling, identifying the problem is an extension of the assessment stage in the nursing process. One of the principal differences is that of diagnosis. Generally speaking, a clinical diagnosis is made by a doctor, who then tells the patient what he thinks is wrong with him. Unlike the doctor, however, the counsellor does not make a unilateral diagnosis; both counsellor and client identify the problem area.

Active involvement

Schein (1969) speaking of process consultation within organizations (a process similar to counselling) in contrast to the doctor–patient model says, "What is wrong, of course, is that the doctor, the consultant, has not built up a common diagnostic frame of reference with the patient, his client. If the consultant does all the diagnosis while the client—the manager—waits passively for a prescription, it is predictable that a communication gulf will arise which will make the prescription seem irrelevant and/or unpalatable." This warning is salutary for all who work with other people. There are many patients who ignore the treatment prescribed by their doctors because what they received was not what they went for. Schein goes on to say "... the client must learn to see the problem for himself, to share in the diagnosis and to be *actively involved* in generating a remedy ... a key role in helping to sharpen the diagnosis and in providing alternative remedies which may not have occurred to the client". This is exactly the aim of counselling where the client is encouraged to make his own decisions and to stand by them (with help from the counsellor if necessary), if they prove to be the wrong ones. Another aim is that by helping the client solve his immediate problem, he will be given encouragement to solve future problems without aid from the counsellor.

The shift in emphasis from a unilateral assessment to a joint activity, which Schein suggests and which counsellors endorse, may not always be an easy manoeuvre to make, particularly for those people who have been accustomed to making or accepting clinical diagnoses. But so fundamental is it to counselling that it cannot be overstressed just how important it is that the client feels genuinely involved in the process.

Confidentiality

Confidentiality was touched on in Chapter 2, when the idea of a contract was discussed. In the early stage of meeting the client it is desirable to bring this topic into the open. The client may have some vague idea that nothing he says will be in confidence, particularly if counselling takes place within an institution, such as a hospital. On the other hand, he may think that absolutely everything will be a closely guarded secret. That is one reason why it is essential, when making notes, that the use to which they will be put is explained. It is also necessary to explain the role of the mentor (as discussed in Chapter 2). Elsewhere a distinction is made between material that is 'confidential' and that which is secret (Stewart 1977). It is essential to discriminate between the two. It may be necessary, when counselling a patient, that some record be made in his notes. But such a record need not contain every detail of the discussion. The nurse must make a conscious decision what to include and what to omit.

> Mr Carlos, in the course of counselling, revealed that he had a criminal record. The nurse decided that this information, if withheld, would not affect the treatment. She did not include this detail in the notes, but concentrated on Mr Carlos's anxiety about his forthcoming exploratory operation for cancer.

> Mrs Angus, being treated for varicose veins, revealed that her husband was, in fact, not her legal husband. The nurse felt that there was no necessity to include this detail.

> Mrs Steptoe, when she was being interviewed, on one of her frequent admissions for ulcerative colitis, let slip that her husband had disappeared some 10 years previously. From the way she told her story, and the fact that her first admission was almost 1 year after his disappearance, the nurse did include this in her write-up and discussed it with the doctor. Mrs Steptoe had agreed that the nurse disclose this information. She was reluctant at first, lest the police become involved, but when the doctor spoke with her and reassured her that this would not be so, she was able to talk to the nurse much more freely about her feelings. Through exploration of her feelings, she was able to see how her anxieties had possibly had some bearing on her medical condition.

If the nurse feels that information given by the client should, in his interests, be passed on, this should be discussed fully with him. Most people will agree when it is pointed out to them why it is to be done. However, there could be some who, in spite of all logical reasoning, still refuse permission to disclose. In the end, it is the nurse who must decide, basing her decision on the questions "What may happen if I do disclose it against the client's will?" and "What may happen if I do not disclose it?" If, on balance, she decides that to disclose it against the client's will would so seriously damage the relationship she has with him that further counselling would be jeopardized, she may decide against disclosure. This is a delicate balance to maintain, and being able to do so comes with experience, backed up by having a reliable mentor with whom to discuss the dilemma, still maintaining confidentiality, and without naming the client.

A different situation may arise when the client blurts out his story, then says, "Now, what I've told you is in confidence. You won't tell anyone else, will you?" What he may mean is, "Don't tell the chap in the next bed, my neighbours, the police, my wife." He may *not* mean, "Don't tell those who need to know; those who are reliable and responsible for my treatment." A person who says this—either before or after a disclosure—is really presenting an ideal opportunity to discuss the whole question of confidentiality. At all costs, avoid being trapped into giving a sweeping guarantee of absolute confidentiality, especially before hearing what is involved. Establish clearly and precisely what the client means.

Stage 2 skills

The skills outlined in the previous chapter continue throughout counselling, but in later stages these skills acquire new emphases. Listening, for example, becomes more active and directed. It is not uncommon for the client to repeat something he has previously related. There are a number of reasons for this. The principal one is that at first telling it did not register with him that he had told it. Therefore, he needs time to retell it. It is also very likely that since the previous telling, new thoughts have come to him which he needs time and space to explore. What is equally important is that at the first telling he may not have been able to attach the appropriate feelings to the words. Now, having had time for the emotions to settle, he feels the need to match words to feelings. It is also possible that at the first telling, the nurse did not hear the feelings being expressed; he is thus giving her another chance. Another possibility is that at the time, he and the nurse were not in complete rapport, so the message was not sensitively received. That is why, in the later stages, listening assumes a fresh importance.

Reflecting

Here the nurse reflects back to the client (as does a mirror) the factual content of on the one hand, what he is saying, and, on the other, the feelings *as she perceives them.* She should never assume that her perceptions are always accurate. Any reflection of feeling must be tentative. "You said that you were told you were going to be made redundant a week before it happened, and this knocked the bottom out your world, is that it?" This is focusing on the facts but linking the feelings to them. "You're giving me a very strong impression of still being depressed about your mother's death, would that be right? Even though, as you said, it was 2 years ago."

Not only may the nurse reflect the facts and feelings by putting them into her own words, she may use the same words as the client used. This has the effect of letting him hear them again and hearing them may release feelings hitherto held in check.

Mary was talking to Peter about his relationship with his boss.

Mary: You say he's an absolute pig to work for, is that right?
Peter: I didn't say that, did I? What a horrible thing to say about
            someone. I may have thought it.

This led to a fruitful discussion of how so often our lips say what our hearts mean.

If reflecting is like looking in a mirror, caution must be exercised, for a mirror may so easily distort, particularly if there is a flaw in it. It must also be remembered that the mirror-image is the reverse of the true. That is why reflections must be tentatively offered, and having offered them, the client may reject them if he is unable to identify with them.

Another aspect of reflecting is linking what the person is saying with what he is doing, or has done.

You say you don't mind your wife having this friendship with another man, that it is only platonic, but every time you mention this man, your fists clench, as if you were angry. Is that worth looking at?

If the client has given a lengthy statement, it may not always be easy to pick up a central issue and this may leave the listener feeling swamped. It is probably better not to try to hold on to every detail, but to comment on the last part, assuming that if the client stops speaking he has done so because he is now ready for some feedback. If the statement has been overlong, leaving the nurse confused, she could make a positive contribution by saying how she feels, "… and I'm not at all sure which thread to pick up". This may have the effect of causing the client to do some self-reflecting. But even where it is difficult to pick up a specific feeling on which to comment, it may be possible to reflect how the statement was made. "That seemed very long and complicated and you seemed under great pressure to talk.

Was that because of ...?" may be as helpful as anything more profound. This leads quite naturally to the next skill.

Paraphrasing

Paraphrasing, according to one dictionary definition, is "a free rendering or an amplification of a statement". It may condense or it may expand the words used. In general conversation many assumptions are made about what has been said. Counselling is not an 'ordinary' conversation. Both nurse and client constantly need to be sure that they understand each other; paraphrasing helps to ensure this.

Words are vehicles to convey feelings. So not only is it necessary for the nurse to understand the client's words, she must also try to understand why particular words, in preference to others, are used. If the client has been expressing his thoughts with difficulty, then is a good time to paraphrase. Letting him hear the meaning from someone else's lips not only provides an opportunity to hear it in this way, but also demonstrates that the nurse is really attending. Paraphrasing, well done, encourages the client to continue.

An aspect of paraphrasing is seeking clarification. A simple "I don't understand that bit" helps the client to be more precise. If he seems unable to clarify what he means, restating may be all that is required. It may help him, in a particularly difficult blockage, for the nurse to use an illustration or an analogy. If possible, these should be within the client's experience; this is likely to be more telling than if they arise purely out of the nurse's experience.

Joe, a bricklayer, during counselling over his difficulty in maintaining satisfactory relationships with girlfriends, experienced a blockage as Alice was encouraging him to look at his contribution to the breakdown.

Alice: When you are building a wall, where do you start?
Joe: At the foundation, of course.
Alice: And then?
Joe: You build it up, brick by brick.
Alice: And what holds the bricks together?
Joe: Cement.
Alice: I expect you can build a wall in a day, can you?
Joe: Not if it's a big wall, no. It will take time. I'll have to stop to take measurements and make sure it's straight. No, it's hard work

and can't be hurried. I've got to be patient and use all my
skill. (Here there was a long pause, which Alice was in no
hurry to interrupt.) You are crafty, aren't you! That's what
I'm not doing with my friends. I'm not prepared to take time
to get to know them properly. I've got to learn to build.

They then entered into a fruitful discussion of what the bricks in a
relationship were and the cement that bound them together, yet kept them
apart.

Summarizing

Summarizing, like paraphrasing, when well done is not an intrusion, but it
should not be overdone. Summarizing may occur at any time during a
session and is useful to highlight recurring themes. When Alice first met
Joe, she was struck by the way he related a series of broken relationships.
Her question, "Have all your relationships with girls ended in disaster?"
was a useful summary of what had been a long tale of woe and self-pity.

A summary at the end of a session is essential for several reasons. It gives
the client an opportunity to hear again the main points; it gives the nurse an
opportunity to clarify and consolidate her understanding of what has taken
place; it provides an opportunity for both, and particularly the client, to
think about the next session.

Specificity

Getting the client to be specific may be quite difficult; it is an art that
requires much practice. But it is essential if he is to come to terms fully with
whatever is causing him concern. Specificity covers three areas: what is
said; feelings; and experience. The opposite of specific is 'general' and so
often the client will escape into generalities and vagueness. A generality,
common in everyday speech, is 'you'. The client who says "You never know
when people approve of what you're doing", when encouraged to rephrase
it to "I never know when people approve of what I'm doing", will usually be
able to perceive it in a different light. Personalizing it in this way makes it
pertinent and real. In one sense, this is similar to 'owning the problem'.
Being specific opens the way for a realistic acknowledgement of feelings.

Some people have the tendency to attribute feelings and behaviour to
other people: 'them', 'they', 'us' instead of 'I', 'me'. Having said this,
however, it is often very difficult to break habits of long standing. The

person who always depersonalizes feelings by attributing them to other people may find great difficulty saying, "I feel angry, hurt, sad".

Another part of encouraging the client to be specific is when he is relating some aspect of his behaviour. "I always get into great panics" is a general statement. "Give me a specific example" would encourage him to cut through his tendency to generalize. A possible reason why there is this tendency is to do with owning feelings that are somehow thought of as wrong. To say "I feel angry about sexual exploitation of children" is much stronger than "Many people feel angry about the sexual exploitation of children." The latter example has a defusing effect. Owning such feelings, and not merely reporting them, opens the door to exploring them. While this may be uncomfortable for the client, it may be vitally necessary.

A point that ought to be made is that if a statement such as the one on exploitation of children is made early on in counselling, before the relationship has been firmly established, it might be better to ignore it and not attempt to push the client to be specific. The reason why this particular skill is introduced in the second stage is that it does require the client to be prepared to examine himself closely and not to hide behind the façade of generalities. To do this requires confidence, not only in himself, but also in the counsellor.

The client may fiercely resist all attempts to encourage him to be specific, particularly about his feelings. Being able to talk about one's feelings is something not everyone finds easy to do; perhaps not all have learned how. If this is so, the client may need to be led gently into this learning experience. Most people know how anger or sorrow feels but some feelings require much finer tuning. This is where the nurse may adopt a teaching role. It is important, of course, that the nurse recognizes within herself when she evades being specific by escaping into general statements. All the while she colludes with the client by allowing him to talk about feelings second-hand, as if they belonged to other people and not to him, constructive counselling will be limited. "Is that how you feel?" or "Is that something like your situation?" may be enough to bring the interview back into focus from the 'then and there' to the 'here and now'.

Maintaining momentum

During the early stages of counselling, as the nurse and the client are getting to know each other and as the client spends time telling his story, there may not be any pressing need for the nurse to find ways to keep the interview on the move. Later on, however, when the tale has been told and the problem has been identified, or partially so, and as counselling enters the exploratory stage, it may happen that the process slows up or comes to a halt. There are a number of possible reasons for this.

Sometimes the nurse may get the impression of having 'been here before'; not exactly a déjà vu but a certain sense of repetition. A moment's reflection may be enough to reveal that the wheel has come full circle. Then is the time either to move on or to terminate the interview. Perhaps the client has had enough, or perhaps the nurse has. To move the interview on it may be sufficient to say something like, "We seem to have come full circle. Shall we carry on?" If this approach is not used, the nurse may refer to something that emerged earlier in the session, or the client be asked at which point he would like to restart. He may be able to tell why he has come back to the beginning. The nurse, earlier, may have dealt inadequately with the point which has now re-appeared. But it is also possible that only by going back can the client speak about something that caused him difficulty before. It could also mean that the nurse is trying to direct him into an avenue that she felt could have been explored before but was not. If the client does not accept her lead, he may perceive it as a stumbling block which will almost certainly slow down the interaction.

Comments such as "and then?"; "what happened?"; "what was the outcome?"; "tell me about ..."; "what were your feelings at the time?" are all aimed at moving the interview forward—gently, not pushing it. But there is usually a natural time for a session to end. If momentum slows down, that may be the appropriate time to stop, by summarizing what has taken place.

On the other hand, momentum may slow down because the client is thinking deeply about some comment the nurse has made or something that has 'popped' into his mind, possibly triggered off as part of a chain reaction. He may be hesitating to mention something, not certain of its relevance, its importance or possibly its controversial nature. The nurse may have become preoccupied, allowing her attention to waver. When this happens, the client will feel uneasy; conversation most likely will stop.

Silences

One way of maintaining momentum, although it may seem a paradox, is the constructive use of silence. The silence that comes from blockage has already been mentioned. In that sort of silence, the nurse may be able to help by suggesting something to the client, but the client should be given time to think and also to feel. So often, what could be a constructive silence is ruined by an overanxious counsellor, unable to tolerate the silence, or possibly feeling that the client cannot tolerate it.

Silences may also arise as a result of the interaction between the nurse and the client. Perhaps she has pushed him too far, too quickly, thus causing him alarm. In this instance, silence is a retreat. The client may feel resentful that he is not really being listened to. Perhaps he keeps making a point which the nurse keeps missing. Something the nurse says may set up emotional vibrations which the client finds difficult to handle. Once again, he may retreat into silence. He may feel like saying something critical but does not want to hurt the nurse, so he keeps silent.

Broadly speaking, silences are of two kinds: positive and negative. In the first, the atmosphere is comfortable, like sitting with a friend by a nice log fire, sharing a meal. The other is full of tension and most uncomfortable. In the former, movement forward usually presents no problem. A comment such as "That feels really comfortable. I wonder what was passing through your mind just then?" may well open doors that hitherto have been barred.

With negative silences it may be less easy to get things going again. It depends on what has created the silence. If the nurse feels that she has wittingly or unwittingly caused the silence, she should say so. A moment's reflection may show her the reason. If not, a simple comment, "We've gone quiet and it makes me feel uncomfortable. I've a feeling that something I said has caused it. Am I right?" may prove to be just the thing to get things moving. If the client responds positively, this can provide a useful focus for movement forward. Even if the nurse is unable to think what has caused the silence, taking the 'blame', as it were, may be a productive way of breaking the silence without too much trauma. Silences which are allowed to go on may demoralize both nurse and client.

If the nurse feels that the negative silence arises more from within the client than as a result of her intervention, again she may help to break out of this by a comment such as, "This silence makes me feel ... Are you finding it difficult to put something into words?" This fairly open approach then leaves the client free to choose how he will respond. It is possible that he may not have felt the silence as uncomfortable, and may seem surprised that the nurse did. None the less, this too could lead to a fruitful discussion on feelings. In closing this section on silence, it is worth repeating what was said earlier: do not be in too much of a hurry to break silences; do not feel that every gap in conversation has to be filled immediately with words. Some of the most constructive work is done in silence.

Counselling is like travelling from London to Brighton. It can be done by express train, car, bicycle or on foot. For each of these modes of travel, the pace will be different. Some counselling interviews can proceed at a rapid pace; others are much slower. It is the client who sets the pace. Any attempt to force him to change from a walking pace to a run, in all probability, will result in 'client fatigue'. One client may be quite able to dash along; the nature of his problem and his emotional state may permit him to do this quite happily. Another person may want to walk, so as to view the countryside as it passes. If, somewhere along the road, he decides to hasten his pace, so be it. The skilful counsellor will be able to adapt to this change and still remain alongside the client.

This chapter is drawn to a close by directing attention to the fact that certain medications may interfere with the client's ability to comprehend what is being said to him and how he should reply. He may also have difficulty establishing appropriate emotional contact with the nurse. Specific conditions and how they affect the client's responses are not dealt with in this book, but most people know from their own experiences that when they are anxious or unhappy, their respones are different than at other times. Anyone who has wakened from a drugged sleep (or from an anaesthetic) knows how wooly his thoughts are. Many treatments produce the effect of a certain sense of unreality which makes it difficult for the patient to grasp what he sees and hears. This can produce further anxiety, particularly if he knows that the original difficulty is still there. One patient, who had been on long-term antidepressants, said, "It is like looking at my problem through thick frosted glass; glass that obscures and changes the shape of my problem, but prevents me from getting at it. This worries me a great deal, that it is still there and I can do nothing about it."

So staying alongside the client may not always be easy. In the case just quoted, although not a great deal of exploration of the original problem was possible, much was achieved as the patient was helped to focus on what he felt was happening within him at that moment. This paid dividends; for when the confusion lifted, he had established a sound working relationship with the nurse and together they were able to move on into exploring the problem that had brought him into hospital.

References

Schein, E H (1969) Process Consultation: It's Role in Organization Development, Addison-Wesley, p 7

Stewart, W (1977) A Guide to Counselling: Every Manager a Counsellor, Wessex Regional Health Authority, p 7

CHAPTER 4

EXPLORE THE PROBLEM

Stepping stones not stumbling blocks

Exploration requires great sensitivity and skill. The aim is to help the client explore different aspects of whatever problem is confronting him. It is probably the most difficult stage. It is also the most delicate. It is so easy to cross the line between genuine exploration and blatant nosiness. In this stage it is possible, by trying too hard, to put stumbling blocks instead of stepping stones in the path of the client. In this stage, where unknown territory often has to be trodden, the nurse has to be more aware of the client's need for empathic support during times when exploration may be difficult or traumatic. From the nurse's point of view, it is here where she herself is most likely to feel in need of the support of a mentor, particularly where exploration is slow. This applies especially to on-going counselling, when discouragement may become very real to both her and the client.

Opening doors

During the previous stage of identifying the problem, the client may have reached a new understanding of what his problem really is. As together they have looked at some possible avenues, light may have begun to shine through some of the chinks which have been created. Now it is time to knock on a few doors and explore what lies beyond.

Counselling is like being in a large room with many doors. As they converse, the nurse may become aware that the client seems to be heading in a certain direction, but before he can proceed there is a door through which he must pass. The nurse puts her hand on the door (figuratively) and may say something like, "It looks as if you mean this", or "Is this what you feel you want?" If this is done sensitively, without a sudden throwing wide of the emotional door, the client then has the opportunity to accept or reject what has been said or suggested. He will, by his response, make it plain whether or not he is emotionally ready, and this is a vital step in counselling. The nurse allows the door to open a bit more, almost as if to permit him a glimpse of what lies beyond. If this stage is moved through gradually, the client, with the nurse alongside, will pass through to take a closer look. This does not mean that all will be revealed. For just as in a house that has remained unoccupied for some time, there may be dust sheets to be removed in order to reveal what lies beneath. The nurse must not expect that all the emotional dust sheets will be removed. The client may not feel the need to look at what lies hidden. That is his prerogative and he must be allowed and encouraged to exercise his freedom of choice. He must do the uncovering. If he is not emotionally ready, any forced or precipitate uncovering may cause him not only to reject what he sees, but also to reject any further counselling.

Within this room there may well be some emotional paraphernalia which are only glanced at in passing, as it were. Others may never be looked at, because they are not recognized, not considered significant or possibly because the client intuitively feels that to expose what lies beneath the dust sheets would be too painful. The nurse, by virtue of her experience, may well detect the presence of items of which the client seems unaware. It is possible that when a person either does not see or decides not to look, that at some time in the future, when other things have prepared the way, he may feel the need to re-enter that particular room and continue exploring where he left off.

This process of opening doors and examining the contents which lie beyond may be repeated many times, as different doors are opened. But there are likely to be some doors, at least during counselling, which remain firmly barred against entry. Counselling does not necessarily involve probing into the deep recesses of the dim and distant past. Past and present are bound together but counselling is more concerned with the present and the very recent past. Exploration of the emotions of the present frequently opens doors to the emotional contents of the past. The client, to come to terms with the past, may need to explore them within the present counselling relationship.

Exploration—a dual activity

It should be emphasized that exploration is very much a dual activity, involving both client and nurse. This has already been intimated in the analogy of the doors. Sometimes the client may lead the way; at others it is the nurse who will move in a certain direction, always realizing that such leading is tentative. She must be ready to retreat the instant she becomes aware that she is no longer alongside the client. Leading in this way must be done very gently. It must be leading, not pushing; in no sense must she give the impression that she knows the way to go. Unlike other forms of exploration, there are no maps of any certainty. Previous journeys only point the general direction. They do not, indeed cannot, provide every detail. What was significant for one client may have no significance whatever with another. That is why each client opens up new and exciting areas for discovery.

Broadly speaking, the nurse sets out to help the client explore significant areas in his life, as well as the significant people. It is also necessary to help him explore how these areas and people interact with each other. For example, Alexander, married with children and parents still alive, worked in a factory. He also had a part-time job as a barman in a public house and he played string bass in a jazz group. He had a health problem in that he had been having tachycardia. One way of helping him to explore what seemed like a fairly formidable list would be:

Significant people	*Significant areas*
Wife	Work
Children	Part-time work
Parents	Group
Workmates (factory and pub)	Health
Group	

Exploration revealed that he had the part-time job and played in the band because his wife could not manage the household budget effectively. The children were noisy and unruly (he blamed his wife but she says that he is hardly ever at home). So he escapes by becoming involved in outside activities. He detests his work and would prefer to be a full-time musician, but he feels trapped in domesticity. He regards tachycardia as a sure indication that he is going to die young.

The nurse working with him helped him to see possible links between these different factors which created a picture of someone whose present medical condition may have been influenced by his way of life. As they explored these various strands, she was conscious that he was unwilling to enter into any exploration related to his parents. Several times she 'led' him towards this door. The third time he said, "You obviously want me to talk about my parents. I don't want to. Please leave it there." Not all clients will be as forthright as he was, but at least the nurse knew that no useful purpose would be served by pursuing this. Counselling may not always produce neat answers.

Self-awareness

It could be said that the general aim of counselling is to increase the client's self-awareness and insights and to marshal these new-found strengths in working towards an action plan that will help him to cope more effectively with life. It could be cogently argued that even if insight is achieved, this alone is not sufficient for some clients to cope. Some clients need a great deal of sound practical support and guidance in order to cope with life. But, at the same time, sound practical support, unless it is matched with understanding and insight, may be disregarded. Such was the case of Alexander. He had visited his general practitioner who said "You are overdoing it. Something must go." Alexander could not accept this sound practical advice, but as the nurse helped him explore the relationship between significant areas and people, insight came. "I suppose I'm doing all these things to escape from a home where I don't feel a great deal of love. Yet, in reality, if I go on like this I'll end up possibly not able to work at all. Then I'll really feel that I'm in prison." As a result of talking it through, he decided to give up the jazz band, the activity he considered the most stressful.

Stage 3 skills

Here and now: then and there

In stage 2, the nurse may have used specificity to encourage the client to be explicit. In stage 2, she may want to use another skill—here and now—to look at the interaction between herself and the client. Counselling can quite usefully be regarded as a role-modelling relationship. Although it is not the intention to mould clients into counsellors, there is little doubt that where clients have sustained contact with counsellors, many of them do pick up and use some of the ways of responding to people. Clients who have experienced difficulty in being open, for example, frequently end up being able to talk more freely about their feelings. And, what is more, they are often able to help other people to do likewise.

Thus, the nurse has an ideal opportunity when counselling to use the relationship in a positive way. In stage 3 much more use is made of 'self'—the nurse as a person—to focus attention on interaction. Some clients, like those who generalize and need help to be specific, may be helped to examine what is actually happening in counselling. Clients who have a tendency to talk about feelings *in the past*, rather than now, may be helped if the nurse can point to something in the 'here and now'— something that is happening between them—to help identify present feelings. As specificity contrasts with generality, so 'here and now' contrasts with 'then and there'. The principal difference is that in the one the client is encouraged to own his feelings and not to generalize; in the other, he is encouraged to own his feelings as they exist *at that moment*. At the same time, the nurse herself may show the way by talking of her feelings in the interaction.

When Alexander was talking to his counsellor, she said, "When you talk about your wife, you sound as if you're talking about a little child. Just now you used the same sort of tone to me. I felt really very small." This brief exchange helped Alexander to realize that in his relationships he often treated women in this way. In other words, the nurse used how she felt to help him see that other people could possibly feel the same way.

People who always talk of events and feelings in the past and never in the present, may be helped to do so by a comment such as, "I find it difficult, listening to you, to know how you really feel right now. Everything seems so remote." This almost forces the client to face how he does feel *at that moment*. He may feel angry, surprised or hurt at this suggestion. But that reaction can be used effectively to demonstrate the difference between the here and now and then and there. It is worth stressing again that if the nurse is able to use what is happening between them, to point to what may happen between the client and other people, a great deal will have been accomplished.

Self-disclosure

Self-disclosure means that the nurse decides to reveal something of herself to the client. Disclosure must be used with discretion. Not that the client may misuse what the nurse reveals, but that inappropriate or mistimed disclosure may increase rather than decrease the client's anxiety. Accurately used, however, self-disclosure can be positive and helpful and assist in reducing the aura of omnipotence that sometimes surrounds counsellors.

The occupational-health nurse working with Peter Treadmill (see p. 46), who disclosed that she too had experienced the trauma of coping with a severely mentally handicapped child, was disclosing a very sensitive part of herself. It may have been disadvantageous if she had dwelt overlong on her own feelings. To do so would have removed the focus from Peter. Removing the focus may be one of the reasons why counselling loses momentum.

Not all counsellors agree about self-disclosure. There are those who never give any information about themselves, believing that to do so would get in the way of constructive counselling. Injudicious disclosure most certainly may, but if it is done sensitively and with the motive of helping the client deal with some feeling, it can be productive.

One of the dangers of self-disclosure, apart from removing the focus by undue attention to the facts and feelings presented by the counsellor, is the impression that may be given of "If I have overcome it ..." or "this is what I did ...", the implication being that the client can do likewise.

Sheila, a third year student nurse, asked her tutor for 'advice'. She had become involved with a married man and was having difficulty coping with the emotional upheaval within her. Hardly had she finished the brief introduction, when the tutor said, "I know how you feel, Sheila. The same thing happened to me. What I did was to get a transfer to another school to complete my training. That was how I coped. Perhaps you could think along those lines." Sheila felt that her time was being wasted, so excusing herself she left, feeling sore and frustrated. Very soon after this, she discontinued training for 'personal reasons'.

This may have happened in any event, but the fact that she was not really listened to must have influenced her decision. In this instance, self-disclosure, no doubt done with the best of intentions was inappropriately used to control the interview and not to permit exploration of Sheila's feelings. Inappropriate self-disclosure may be used in an attempt to create rapport. It may also be used for self-gratification by the nurse who wants to talk about her own life, rather than listen to the client.

Confrontation

Confrontation is not fisticuffs! There are times when it is wiser to ignore than to comment, but there are also times when it could be valuable for the client to know how the nurse feels about some part of the interaction. This is one aspect of confrontation that is similar to the 'here and now' interaction. Another is where the client may benefit from being confronted with the possible outcome of his behaviour or some contemplated course of action. In this sense, confrontation is helping him look at reality, or at least at reality as seen through the eyes of the nurse. If confrontation is not physical fisticuffs, neither is it verbal fisticuffs. Any confronting is best put in a tentative way, as a suggestion, rather than as a statement of fact and then only after careful deliberation. It should never be used as a retaliation.

When Andrew met Jane, she was having problems getting to work on time. "I'm always tired and I sleep in." During the session it emerged that she had strong religious views, which to Andrew's mind did not correspond to her seeming lack of responsibility towards her job. He said, "You speak of your religious principles: how do these tie up with often arriving late?" She looked startled, saying, after some hesitation, "Not very well. It's not a good witness, is it?" Andrew felt that nothing more needed to be said at that moment. They then went on to look at how this pattern of behaviour might be changed.

If Andrew had said, "I don't think your religious principles match up with your behaviour", Jane could have felt under attack. She may have retreated; she may have retaliated.

The aim of confrontation is certainly not to make the client feel small, nor to 'get at him'. If it is carried out with as much respect, interest and understanding as any other part of counselling, filtered through caring, it will usually be well received. It is better, if possible, to focus on some aspect of behaviour than on some aspect of personality. This is what Andrew did, though he did link Jane's behaviour to something in her personality. He could have put it as "Do you see any conflict in often arriving late?" and let her work through to what he had in mind. But as he said later, "She seemed pretty complacent about it all. What I did (though not consciously calculated) was to give her a jolt and shake her out of her complacency."

Finally, confrontation is generally only used when the relationship is firmly established. If the client is not certain of the nurse, he may perceive her comment (valid though it might be) as an unwarranted attack. The other side of this is that the nurse must know the client well enough to make a judgement of how confrontation will be received.

Penetration

Feelings may be identified at various levels. It is quite likely that in the early stages of counselling, the nurse will be involved mainly with the client's superficial feelings. But as counselling progresses, she will invariably have to help him get at feelings that lie beneath the surface. Normally, getting in touch with deeper feelings can only be achieved as the nurse and client begin to establish a mutually empathic understanding and as the nurse demonstrates that she is aware of how the client is feeling—sad, anxious, fearful, angry, happy, excited, and so on.

The principal difference between exploration of superficial feelings and penetration to deeper ones is that quite often superficial ones are expressed without too much hesitation; deeper ones often remain unstated. The client may be dimly aware that they are there but needs help to make them explicit.

The client who is experiencing difficulty in trying to decide what to do with her home now that her husband is dead and her children have all married may need help to accept the fact that her true problem is one of loneliness.

To another client one might say, "You say that you didn't want to come into hospital because it made you feel helpless. You also said that you had been in hospital as a child. Is there any connection with the way you feel now and the way you felt then?"

Penetration is generally best approached with a phrase such as, "I wonder if ...", "Do you think that ...?" "It seems possible that what you're really saying (or feeling) could be ..." It is always useful to ask, "How does that sound to you?" Feelings may be so easily misinterpreted.

Extrapolation

This is where the nurse encourages the client to look beyond the immediate. It may be a looking back or a looking forward. By the client putting himself in different situations in the future, he can be helped to judge how he may react and feel. Likewise, by relating the past to the present, he may be helped to see that what he did and what he was in the past influenced what he is and does now. Very often it is a case of putting up counselling Aunt Sallys, just for the client to experience knocking them down.

However, at this point it is possible to move from true exploration to pure (though disguised) prying, which then becomes offensive to the client who, because of his circumstances, may be very much a captive audience. If the nurse listens accurately to the client's feelings, she will pick up cues that she is treading on inappropriate ground. On the other hand, it could be appropriate ground, but the timing may be inappropriate.

Advice

The section on extrapolation leads quite naturally into this section on advice. The dictionary defines counsel as advice, yet this one word is an anathema to many counsellors. In its widest sense, and certainly as a lawyer would use it, it is not "do this" but rather "this is what is possible"—an opening up of alternatives and possibilities. In this sense the dictionary definition could be correctly applied to counselling. But, unfortunately, to the word 'advice' has been attached the undesirable meanings of "this is what you should do" or "what you ought to do". In a way, "this is what you should do" is direction and control, and not in legal terms advice. It is unfortunate that advice and advising have become unacceptable words in counselling.

One of the basic assumptions in any counselling is that the person is helped to work towards his own solution. This is why it is important to help him explore as many different avenues as possible; and it is in this area that the concept of advice appears to create conflict. Davison (1965) says, "The way she (the caseworker) presents alternatives or points out the legal consequences of certain actions must give some bias, but, provided that she leaves with the client as much initiative as he is capable of exercising and gives him every opportunity to discuss whatever he wishes, then she does no violence to the principle of self-responsibility". It is this self-responsibility which is implied in the above sentence about the person working towards his own solution. If, as Davison suggests, the nurse severely limits the choices, then the client may well feel constrained. He may feel that there are no other alternatives open to him and attempt to follow what has been fairly strong (though veiled) direction. In other words, because exploration has been limited, the client has responded to 'closed advice' which implies direction, rather than to 'open advice' which implies freedom of choice.

Images

The final skill to be discussed in this chapter is the use of images to help the client get in touch with the feelings of his inner world. In a sense, the reader has been introduced to the use of images in the analogy of counselling as knocking on doors and exploring what lies beyond, and when Alice was talking with Joe (p. 61). What imaging does is to cut through the intellect and release feelings attached to an inner picture. William was talking about feelings of oppression in his head. Donald said, "Can you get a picture of what it looks like?" After some moments meditating, he said, "It's a dried-up walnut, sitting in the middle of my forehead." He continued to concentrate on this image while it gradually became smaller, then disappeared completely.

Sandra was expressing feelings of loneliness, yet she did not seem a lonely person. Her counsellor asked her to try to get a picture. Almost immediately she saw a clearing in the middle of a large dark wood. In the middle of the clearing was a little girl in a green dress, crying bitterly "... my mummy and daddy have gone and left me here". As she watched, the trees turned into cot bars and she was standing in a hospital cot, shaking it and screaming, "I want my mummy, I want my daddy." This image had released a memory of her at about 3 years of age, admitted for a tonsil operation. The feelings of isolation, loneliness and rejection were very powerful and she was able to see a little of how such feelings may have contributed to her feelings of loneliness in adult life.

Like all the skills outlined in the first three stages, imaging must be used sensitively and intelligently and appropriate to the occasion and the client. Images are generally attached to powerful feelings; and powerful feelings, when released, may cause the client to burst into tears. Words then seem totally superfluous. So often, healing comes when blocked channels are cleared.

The nurse who wants to use the particular technique of imaging and fantasy can practise on herself. Close your eyes and sit quietly and comfortably. Choose an age—say when you were 10—and when the first picture emerges, study it intently until it fades, possibly to be replaced by another picture. Some pictures that emerge may not necessarily be what you expect; some may be bizarre. But the great thing is trust your inner self. Something within you will take care of you and will lead you on without harm.

Another exercise is to select a feeling—love for example—and try to get a picture for it. When you have explored that, try another feeling. If you persist in this way, you will become familiar with what is happening within you. You can then use this when dealing with clients as you receive pictures which may relate to them. Never ignore the feeling which a particular client arouses. If this feeling is then put into picture form and put before the client, it may be just what he needs at that moment to help him break through a particularly difficult blockage.

One last illustration must suffice. Sandra (mentioned above) had been talking for some time about her difficulties. Her counsellor who had not been sitting with closed eyes, but who had been using the imaging technique said "I get the impression of a giant whirlpool and you are caught up in it." Sandra was thoughtful, then said "That is exactly how I do feel, though I've never identified it just like that. Yes, I am afraid of being sucked down by my job (as a nurse) and losing my identity. An in order to prevent this happening, I have to keep frantically busy." This led to a fruitful discussion of her fears about being engulfed by her work.

This brings to a close the first part of the book, dealing with the process of counselling. It is not enough to help the client achieve insight. Part of the skill of counselling is helping him marshal his inner resources to live more as he wants it. Some problems can be resolved with counselling help, others cannot. Part of the task of counselling is helping some people cope with situations that cannot be cured. A man who has had his leg amputated will not grow another; that cannot be cured. But he may respond to counselling to help him come to terms with the fact that he will have to accommodate to a very different lifestyle in the future. The woman whose husband has died still has to bear the loss, but counselling may help her cope more effectively with living her life without him.

Part 2 considers ways in which clients may be helped to put into action some of what has previously been talked about.

Reference

Davison, E H (1965) Social Casework, Baillière Tindall

PART 2

THE ACTION

CHAPTER 5

THE ACTION PLAN

Part 2 will concentrate mainly on one case study, using what emerges to point to the various principles and techniques which may be used in counselling. Where it is desirable, because of lack of appropriate material in this case study, points will be illustrated from other cases.

When the client feels sufficiently free from the forces that have been restraining him then, and only then, will he be able to contemplate action. The aim is to help to discover, then harness, his inner resources which have been locked in. Increased self-awareness and insight are often the keys that will release these resources.

The action plan is divided into two stages: thinking about it and carrying it through. Inadequate thinking it through may spell disaster. The client may feel so much better and more able to cope that his enthusiasm and new-found confidence could run away with him, unless the nurse keeps the emotional brake on. That is why a full exploration of the plan is essential. It slows down the pace, but it should not be allowed to drag on too long.

Case study

Living with angina

This is a case study of a successful, self-employed businessman and his family, who live in a pleasant, modern housing estate in Wiltshire. As a result of his clinical condition, the lifestyle of this family is likely to undergo a dramatic change.

The client: Alan Driver, age 38.*
His wife: Ruth, age 38.
Daughter: Linda, age 18.
Son: Raymond, age 14.

Clinical history

Referred on 10 April 1980 for possible by-pass surgery. Seen in outpatients department on 6 June 1980 complaining of precordial pain and breathlessness on exertion since March 1979. Blood pressure was not raised. Surgeon recommended beta-blockers and to continue with Adalat (nifedipine). (It is said that Adalat has a synergistic effect with beta-blockers.) He was started on propranolol 120 mg daily, in divided doses, to be pushed either to the limit or until pain was relieved. Admitted for coronary arteriography in August 1980. Surgery was not recommended, as his coronary arteries and left ventricle were normal. Five weeks before his arteriograph he stopped his beta-blockers; he didn't like taking tablets. He was advised to give up smoking completely and permanently. He gave it up, but when he heard that surgery was not necessary, he started again.

---

*The client and his wife have both given their consent for this case study to be written. The names have been changed.

Social history

Was self-employed for 7 years as an industrial cleaner. Very hard worker, working up to 18 hours a day. Has not worked for 14 months. Now living on capital, plus weekly sickness benefit. Both his wife and Linda work as telephonists. He has tried to restart a business of his own but has not been able to get the permission of the council. Is very bitter about this; claims there is discrimination and favouritism. "They are hammering me into a hole." Also feels bitter at the way the self-employed are penalized when in need of assistance. Contrasts himself with some of his British Leyland friends who have been made redundant and the help they receive. "I don't owe anybody anything. I'm a good boy, I've paid off all my debts." They do not have a mortgage. "Worked round the clock for 6 years to pay it off." Prospect of employment, he feels, is bleak. "Who wants a man in my condition?" They no longer go out to parties. They go out once a week to the pub, but his wife feels anxious when they are out too long. She also feels anxious when she is out without him. He feels guilty when she goes to work, leaving him at home. His eating habits have changed—no dairy foods. Good marital relationship. Sexual relations still enjoyed but there is some degree of anxiety on her part. He has never experienced chest pain during intercourse. Linda understands her father's position, but Raymond cannot really understand why his dad cannot play football anymore, or why he finds it difficult to play a game of clock golf at their favourite leisure centre.

Rachael, the community nurse working with this family, helped them to identify the following—not in order of priority:

Significant people	Significant areas
Alan	Medical condition
Ruth	Attitudes
Linda	Smoking
Raymond	Diet
The council	Work
	The marriage
	Money
	Status
	Relationship with his children

She then applied the model to continue working with them, as they considered the future.

Identify alternatives

In the first stage of the action plan, the nurse helps the client look at ways of coping with his particular difficulty, by talking these plans through with him in an open way. Because she does not pass judgement, or try to force unacceptable solutions on him, the client will be more inclined to look with confidence at various alternatives. At first glance this may look the same as extrapolation, but the main difference is that here the focus of the exercise is the action plan. It is true that in the action-plan stage, extrapolation may need to be used if the alternatives are to be fully explored. This emphasizes how skills blend into each other, just as do the various stages.

One of the significant points that emerges, as this case is studied, is that any model must be flexible enough to allow the client to back-track if it becomes apparent that certain ground was inadequately covered earlier. This is demonstrated quite clearly as Rachael, on more than one occasion, found herself going over ground she thought had been well covered. Sometimes it may be necessary to return to stage 2 and identify or reclarify what the problem is. More often, however, it will be necessary to return to stage 3. It would not be unreasonable to expect that when ways and means of coping are studied, more exploration becomes necessary.

When Rachael asked Alan what he would like to tackle first, he replied, "A job ... That's what's most important to me. I've been out of work all this time, living on sickness benefit. It really is getting me down."

> **Rachael:** Is the lack of money proving difficult?
> **Alan:** No, not really. We've got enough put away. It's the inactivity. It's the feeling of uselessness.

This feeling of uselessness had emerged much earlier and had been discussed. Rachael thought that Alan had come to terms with it.

> **Alan:** I can't. I really can't. I wake up at the same time as I always went out and then my mind starts going through everything I would have been doing.

Rachael considered that it might be helpful to look at ways and means of what work Alan could do. She referred back to an earlier remark about wanting to start up a new business.

Rachael: Did anyone ever suggest a talk with the DRO* at the
            Department of Employment?
Alan: Never heard of him. I'm not disabled. Would he see me?

This brief extract shows that Alan had not fully accepted this his angina
could be disabling. Rachael then spent more time discussing his feelings,
his hopes and fears about his condition and the possible outcome. This is a
feature of counselling; that so often the client needs to express feelings many
times.

As they talked, it was obvious that Alan had a great deal of bitterness and
resentment still smouldering. Rachael wondered if these negative feelings
were getting in the way of moving forward. She did not speak of this to him,
deciding to leave it until later.

One of the things she suggested they might do was to look at what else he
might do to earn a living.

Alan: Whatever it is it mustn't be too stressful. I realize that now
            after our last chat. It wasn't easy to accept that. I'm still a
            young man and I don't want to be a chronic all my life.
Rachael: It looks as if you're beginning to accept that this condition
            might be a handicap.
Alan: I suppose I am. I like the way you put that. You didn't say
            that I was disabled or handicapped, but that the condition
            was a handicap.
Rachael: Yes, that does make a difference. Does accepting it make
            it easier to look at what you might do in the future?

Rachael does not dwell on the fact that her comment has pleased Alan.
She gently pushes him into thinking about future plans.

Alan: I don't really know. Nothing seems to click.
Rachael: Tell me about your hobbies. Perhaps something will
            emerge from that.
Alan: I've never had any time for them. Just an odd game of golf.
            What I am good at is getting business. Perhaps that's
            something I could think about; getting business for other
            people. I needn't do the hard graft—I've had enough of

---

*DRO: Disablement Resettlement Officer.

that. I could act as a sort of agent for industrial cleaning.
I've got the contacts.

Identify goals

Identifying goals which may be achieved soon, if not immediately, and
longer-term ones is a positive approach for the client, who even at this
stage may not see how his problem is to be tackled.

Rachael and Alan sat down and did just that. Rachael was very
conscious how necessary it was to give Alan something positive to work
towards; something that would produce some results. It was obvious that
finding the right type of work would be quite a long-term goal. His
attitude towards smoking and diet would also be long term, though here
she recognized that it would have to be Alan who wanted to change and
not her imposing her standards on him.

She suggested that he make a list of his goals; breaking them down into
short term and longer term. After several minutes, with pencil poised in
hand,

Alan: I can't do it. Apart from getting a job, I can't think of
anything else.
Rachael: Fine. Start there. What do you have to do to get another
job?
Alan: Well, I suppose one of the first things would be to visit
the DRO. Could that be a short-term goal?

By the end of the session, his list looked like this:

Long term	Short term
Get job	See DRO
	Think about agency
Get well again	Stop smoking
	Review eating habits
	Review attitude towards
	medication
Be more at peace	Get rid of resentment and
with myself	bitterness
	Learn to relax

The short-term or enabling goals came only after the long-term ones had been identified. To have left the goal as "I want to get well again" would have been too daunting, too vast and difficult to grasp hold of. In much the same way as it is very difficult to grasp the concept of "working to save the world from starvation".

Rachael: What do you think you could tackle as the easiest of the short-term goals?

Alan: A number of them really. What does strike me, looking at this list, is how much they all interlink. But, as my main preoccupation is getting back to work, maybe I could tackle the DRO first. How do I go about it?

Here Alan is reaching out to Rachael. He seems to have accepted the fact that he does need help, that he is not self-sufficient. This question of self-sufficiency—or being master of one's own ship—was discussed earlier, but for some people it really is a problem. Independence may be a desirable characteristic, but there are some people who rather than control their independence seem to be controlled by it. The fiercely independent person can so easily hurt other people by a thoughtless insistence of "I can manage". It may be more gracious to accept a little help.

Rachael was pleased to hear from Alan that he had visited the DRO. He was sympathetic. At the same time, he was annoyed that no one had thought to mention him to Alan sooner. Although he was considerate, he was not very optimistic about Alan's chances of being able to persuade the council to rent him premises to start up another business. He thought the idea of an agency might be worth pursuing, particularly as Alan's house was large enough to accommodate an office. He did suggest retraining for a job that would not be too demanding, but Alan rejected this. "I've been my own boss for too long", he said. Nevertheless, his visit seemed to put some new spark into him; some new fight that had not been too much in evidence before.

Identify new skills

One of the areas Rachael and Alan looked at was what new skills would he have to acquire to help him achieve his goals? As they examined the idea of an agency, he realized that possibly he would have to cover a much wider geographical area than previously and that with more increase in clientele he would need more sophisticated office skills than he possessed. He would also have to think more about advertising and securing contracts as well as ensuring a good match between client and operator. He found this prospect daunting. Rachael involved Ruth in the discussion. She was employed as a telephonist and although this was a skill she felt she could use, she thought she might be able to retrain in secretarial work and so take over this aspect of the venture. She had discussions with the Department of Employment and was able to enrol on a suitable retraining course. Alan eventually enrolled for a correspondence course on advertising and salesmanship.

Referral

There may be times when the nurse recognizes that she does not possess the skills to deal with a particular client. Rachael was confident that she and Alan and Ruth could work together because Alan's problem had a medical base from which to work. If Alan and Ruth's marriage had not been a stable one, it is possible that Rachael may have felt out of her depth in trying to act as a marriage guidance counsellor, something of which she had no experience. If Alan or Ruth had overt mental instability, again she may have felt unable to cope. If she had come to this realization, she would have been well-advised to suggest to Alan that she find someone else to be his counsellor.

Michael was a community psychiatric nurse to whom Alf was referred. Alf had been admitted to the local psychiatric unit following an attempted suicide. While receiving treatment, it came to light that he also had a drink problem. It was during one of his periodic drinking bouts that he had made the attempt on his life. Michael made contact while Alf was still in the unit. After the first session, Michael reported to his nursing officer, saying that he felt that he did not have the experience of dealing with clients with alcoholic problems. In any case, he did not feel comfortable working with Alf. The nursing officer felt that it would not have been therapeutic for Alf if Michael continued working with him, so he assigned another nurse to work with him. He did not leave it there, however. He encouraged Michael to talk over his feelings about not being able to work with Alf. Michael told him that his own strong views about temperance often seemed to get in the way of understanding the person with alcoholic problems. This was something the nursing officer had not known, but he also realized that Michael had enough insight to know that with such a client he would not feel comfortable, and that rapport and empathy would most certainly be affected. It was left that if Michael felt the need to explore his feelings further, he could do so.

Recognizing one's limitations is a very necessary part of one's professional experience. Inability or refusal to do so could prove harmful to the client and possibly traumatic to the nurse who may find herself swamped and out of her depth. Knowing to whom a client could be referred means that the nurse should be in touch with some one, or some agency, who would be able to advise. Nurses in hospital, as well as those working in the community, would be able to have contact with social workers, who normally would be in a position to advise on which agency or person would be appropriate.

Passing a client on may pose problems for the nurse, as well as for the client. The client will have to re-establish a relationship with another counsellor; the nurse may feel lacking in some way that she had not been able to help this particular client. These feelings are very real and should not be dismissed as trivial, and in a way they are similar to those experienced by counsellors whose clients suddenly stop coming, with no explanation. While it is difficult to measure success in counselling, counsellors would be less than human if they did not feel something when clients terminate abruptly before the agreed time.

One possible reason for this is that counselling may have been nonproductive; the client may feel he is getting nothing out of it. Another reason is that the relationship for that particular client has not been satisfying enough. It could be that the benefits do not outweigh the cost, whatever that means to the client. It could mean that the counsellor has become dissatisfied or discouraged with the progress being made and is giving out messages that she would like to terminate the relationship.

Another reason is one involving feelings. It has been known for clients to express feelings of love for their counsellors. At the same time, they may strongly express negative feelings. This situation has been likened to the parent–child relationship, where both the parents and the child may and frequently do experience strong feelings of like and dislike, love and hate. If clients experience these 'transference' feelings, as they are called, or indeed if the counsellor experiences them in 'countertransference', and if these feelings are not handled constructively, the client may feel in danger of not being able to control them. This may cause him to terminate the relationship prematurely. It may be these countertransference feelings towards the client that cause the nurse to give out messages of "I can't handle this", thus causing him to terminate. If handled constructively (again a trusted mentor is of immense value here) such feelings may provide a useful focus for growth for both client and nurse.

Renegotiate the contract

Having devised the action plan, pointing the way ahead, the client and the nurse may feel that he can now implement the plan without assistance. Some clients may want to try to manage on their own and this may be what they need. For others, the real test would be putting the plan into action and, for them, continuing help may be necessary. In Alan's case, Rachael had agreed in the first instance that she would stay with them until they had "sorted out some of their feelings about Alan's condition and how they were going to proceed". When this stage was reached—when the goals had been identified and the action plan drawn up—she suggested that perhaps Alan and Ruth could now manage without her. This suggestion did not appeal to them; they wanted Rachael to retain some links until they were well on the way to achieving the long-term goals. She agreed to this, but felt that she would have to reduce the frequency of her visits to once a fortnight, with an eventual aim of monthly visits, tailing off even more beyond that. Alan particularly felt that he still needed help with certain points in implementing the plan they had agreed.

CHAPTER 6

IMPLEMENT THE ACTION PLAN

At the close of the previous chapter it was suggested that some clients may decide to implement the plan without assistance. If this is so, the door to future counselling should be left ajar. For in time of difficulty, the client may want a few minutes of the nurse's listening ear to help him over a rough patch—a counselling booster. Some clients, such as Alan, may still need help to bring the plan to fruition.

Information

Before Alan could start to think about putting his plan into action, he needed a great deal of factual information. Some of this has been covered in the previous chapter. It is not suggested that the nurse herself becomes the resource agent for this information. What would be of positive help, however, where the client needs specific help is for them together to locate an information source. The client is then in a position to find out the information for himself. It would have been easy for Rachael to have contacted the DRO on Alan's behalf, but this would have had the effect of removing from him some responsibility for his own decisions and actions. Alan approached the DRO; Rachael was available, should the approach back-fire.

As they worked together to implement the plan, there were many unknown areas on which Alan needed information, particularly on the question of starting an agency. Rachael did not know all the legal and business avenues, but because she was there, she helped Alan think about them in a logical way. He was the sort of man who 'thought on his feet' and when Rachael suggested that he put things on paper, he found this difficult. One of the things she did was to get him to make a list of 'for' and 'against' the idea of an agency. She encouraged him to talk with many people—bank manager, Inland Revenue inspector, the council, other business people, his old clients—to get their opinions which were added to the list. Doing this, although difficult, was rewarding, in that he very quickly appreciated that this helped him to be much more objective about the whole idea. What emerged from this exercise was a very strong 'yes'. He was encouraged to proceed.

Achieving the goals

So far as the first goal went—to get a job—the plan was succeeding. Alan's correspondence course, though not easy, was stimulating. Studying had revealed qualities and strengths he had not known were there. Ruth's secretarial course did not prove quite so successful. She did not really get the hang of typing and although she completed the course, she felt that typing was not for her. What she did gain was a good understanding of office practice which she thought could be used in the agency.

Alan's next goal—"to be more at peace with myself"—was influenced very much by the movement towards his first goal. He was still very impatient at times and when he became impatient, he became anxious. Accompanying his anxiety, some remnants of his resentment, frustration and bitterness were resurrected. Rachael helped him deal with these feelings by allowing him to express them and at times she was conscious of how necessary it was to allow him to express his feelings in this way. What they did notice was that his periods of frustration were becoming fewer and they did not last as long. He became quite skilled at recognizing and acknowledging his feelings, by paying attention to what was happening to him physically. He no longer had to take his pulse to gauge what his heart was doing. He could very quickly assess its rate and the degree of tension, and he came to know that if he did not do something about it immediately, he would feel unwell.

Rachael thought that some form of relaxation would prove helpful, so she arranged for a remedial therapist to teach him deep relaxation and how to release localized tension. This was not an easy skill for Alan to master. His inner tension very often worked against, rather than with, the therapist, but they persevered.

Some of the other goals were less easy to achieve. His smoking remained a problem to him, in spite of his repeated promises to give it up. He was never able to give it up completely, but he did reduce his consumption. He did not find it difficult to cut down on his alcohol. He and Ruth had never had alcohol in the home; for him drinking had been a social occasion at the local pub. He realized that he could no longer tolerate alcohol. His diet was controlled by Ruth who kept strictly to the diet recommended by the doctor.

Agencies and sources

As with information, Rachael was able to point Alan in the direction of certain agencies where specialist help could be obtained; some have already been mentioned. One other agency, which was appropriate in Alan's case, was the British Heart Foundation. Alan made contact with them and although there was no group which met locally, they sent him some useful literature. This was particularly helpful for in it he could read how other people lived and coped with the same condition.

Other clients may need to be put in touch with other agencies, specific to their circumstances. One agency that usually is able to offer assistance is the Citizens' Advice Bureau.* Some areas have established special units that are able to provide information about organizations that are available to assist specific clients.† Another obvious source of information is the

---

*Appendix A.
†Appendix B.

local Social Services Department.* The Department of Health and Social Security† and the Community Health Council‡ will both provide advice and information on a wide range of topics, and they would be able to point the client in an appropriate direction to receive help.

Problem solving

Counselling, within the context of this book, is based on a problem-solving model. While Rachael was still working with Alan, Raymond asked "Could I speak with you privately?" His father raised a questioning eyebrow, but obligingly left the room. After some hesitation, Raymond started to speak about his wish to leave school as early as possible and start work.

Raymond: Mum and Dad are very good, but I can see that Dad won't be his old self again. I want to be out earning my keep. There's no point in staying on at school, is there?

Rachael: You sound as if you've been doing some deep thinking about your future and what responsibility means.

Raymond: I hadn't looked at it like that, but yes, I suppose so. Do you mean that I would be taking on more responsibility, or less, if I left school? I'm a bit confused.

Rachael spent some considerable time with him, after which he thought it would be a good idea if his parents were involved in the discussion. Rachael could see that Alan particularly was not happy with Raymond's proposal and the more they talked, the more frustrated Alan became. Not wishing to leave them in a 'stew', she thought that some of the heat could be taken out of the situation by getting them to look at a structured way of solving problems.

She drew up some questions§ for them, suggesting that mother and father work together and Raymond work on his own. When they had all finished, then they could compare notes. When she next met them, she was delighted to discover a much less tense atmosphere. They had worked out their respective answers and in discussion had arrived at the conclusion that if Raymond wanted to leave school, he should do so, but not because he

---

*Appendix C.
†Appendix D.
‡Appendix E.
§See Appendix F for a full list of questions.

felt he had to. They had talked quite openly for the first time about their financial affairs. This helped Raymond to see that things were not as desperate as he had imagined. Some time later, Raymond decided that he would leave school but only when he had taken and passed at least five 'O' levels.

Decisionmaking

Another useful model is force-field analysis.* This is a decisionmaking technique designed to help an individual understand the various internal and external forces which influence the way he makes decisions. For most of the time these forces are in relative balance; but when something disturbs the balance, decisions are more difficult to make. Having identified the forces, the next stage is to devise strategies to help him reach his goal. For a more detailed description of the model, refer to Appendix G.

Relationships

Throughout this book a great deal of emphasis has been placed on the counselling relationship. This relationship is not an end in itself; it is a means to an end. It would be arrogant to think that the relationship between counsellor and client is the only relationship which the client finds positive and helpful. There are those for whom, although counselling may help to resolve some difficulty, the relationship component may not be significant.

There are other people for whom relationships create problems. For them, counselling is likely to focus on some aspect of relationship and interaction between people. In an earlier chapter, Alice and Joe were introduced. As they worked together, Joe came to realize that not only did he try to rush things, he also warned people off, not just girls, by his possessive attitude. While he was in counselling, he met another "super girl, she seems just right". So great was his enthusiasm that Alice smiled.

Alice: She seems just perfect, doesn't she?
Joe: (with slight hesitation) Yes. You seem to be laughing at me.
Alice: (laughing) It was your bubbling enthusiasm, I think. It seems to carry you away. Is it always like this?

*The force-field analysis model presented here is adapted from the ideas contained in 'A Handbook of Structured Experiences for Human Relations Training', Vol. 11, University Associates Publishers and Consultants, 7596 Eads Avenue, La Jolla, CA 92037, U.S.A.

Joe: Yes, I suppose I am like that. Perhaps there's a danger. Maybe I don't look for faults. Everything has to be perfect.

As they discussed this point, Joe came to see that one of his weaknesses was that because he desperately wanted a friendship, he consistently filtered out any faults and failings of the other person. Alice was able to help him adopt a more realistic approach to other people. One of the things that happened was that because he was virtually blind to faults, when something dramatic did happen, he felt let down and he could not maintain the relationship. It seemed that if the other person could not be perfect, then the relationship had to end. In the course of time, the relationship with that girl did break down, but not before Joe had been able to tolerate, in her, some degree of less than perfection. Eventually Joe did develop a successful relationship with a girl whom he married based on a much more realistic evaluation. Within the counselling relationship he had learned what it was to be realistic, to have realistic expectations of people as they are. This helped him not to be so possessive. He came, albeit slowly, to the realization that his possessiveness arose from a deep-seated fear of losing friendships. "If I hold on to her tightly, she won't run away" was replaced by "I must allow her to run, if she wants to. I hope she doesn't. We have to work hard at making it work."

Humour

Most people have developed techniques for hiding their feelings from other people. Laughter may be one such technique.

Frank, a good-looking nurse teacher, was popular with his students. He was a good teacher, patient, kind and thoughtful. He had been married to Jean for 12 years. He was talking to John, one of his colleagues.

Frank: (laughing while he said) Funny thing happened. I told Jean that you and I were arranging an evening out for some of the students, and before I could finish, she said "There you go, running after those girls again. You see a lot of them, don't you?" I just laughed, not thinking she was serious; but she was.

John: She sounded jealous.

Frank: (laughing) Yes, funny, isn't it. Nothing to be jealous about.

John: Some women are like that. My wife often says much the same thing. Perhaps they all get jealous.

Some days later, John approached Frank.

John: When you were talking about Jean the other day, I don't think I really heard your feelings. You treated it as a bit of a joke, but I did wonder if Jean's remark had hurt you more than you showed. Your laughter put me off.

Frank: You're right, John. I often do this. I don't show my feelings readily. And I know that laughter is a cover-up. Yes, it did hurt. And what made matters worse was that a couple of them sent me birthday cards and when I came into class on Valentine's Day there was a great big card on the desk. I took it home and laughingly showed it to Jean. That sparked off another storm.

John: Why do you think she is reacting like this?

Frank: She doesn't trust me, that's obvious.

John: Could she be afraid?

Frank: Afraid that I might run off with one of them? I hadn't thought of that. Yes, perhaps she is.

Feelings may be filtered through a façade of joviality.

Pain in counselling

Working in the area of relationships sometimes may be painful. There are times when the person doing the counselling may be hurt by clients who break off the relationship prematurely. A natural outcome of this would be self-questioning and possibly self-doubt. On the other hand, and more often than not, counselling is rewarding and satisfying for both client and counsellor. Clients often experience an upsurge of their feelings, particularly as they enter the exploratory stage. It is not that exploration is intended to produce pain, but so often hurt feelings, deeply buried, may be revealed which may reawaken the original pain. But this may be necessary, if healing from within is to take place. Sometimes when a client is exploring some aspect of his feelings, he unconsciously touches something within the counsellor, some deeply hidden trigger-spot.

Susan and Betty were talking in the office (not counselling) about Betty's mother who had died many years before. Before Susan knew it, her eyes had filled with tears and she recalled her own mother's death some 4 years before. This is the sort of thing that can happen so easily in counselling.

When it does, a wonderful opportunity is provided for the nurse to re-examine that particular area of her life, and reach a greater understanding of her own reactions. How she reacts could very well provide some clues as to things in her experience which she has not fully accepted; possibly some area where healing has not been completed.

Practical assistance

Rachael was able to provide Alan with a great deal of practical assistance: help in filling in application forms, drawing up lists of various kinds and acting as a sounding board for his plans. Another counsellor was involved with a client who went to pieces whenever she had to speak on the telephone. This cost her many good jobs for which she was academically qualified. She was much worse when speaking to men. As the counsellor was a woman, she arranged for a male colleague to play various telephone roles. This helped the client's confidence which was boosted so much that she was successful in gaining a coveted position. Counselling therefore may not always consist only of deep psychological exploration. If a practical solution will suffice, the nurse must be prepared to move out with the client to search for that solution.

Support

The client may need a great deal of support while he is implementing the action plan. To draw an analogy from nursing: a patient who has just been diagnosed as having diabetes may be so relieved that at last an answer has been found, that he may not fully appreciate the prospect of a lifetime of injections. But as days pass into months, discouragement and frustration often set in as he struggles to keep his insulin level stable. This means that a great deal of support is essential. Support means understanding, kindness, caring; being there when needed. In a counselling sense, support means making oneself available to listen and possibly to help the client with a particular stage of the action plan. Support for a couple with marriage difficulties meant that William was there to listen to each one of the family as they poured out their feelings when it became evident that the marriage was no longer workable. Support also meant, "Help us, William, to tell the children." Support was helping the children talk about their feelings of being torn in their love for both parents. Support, in another situation, may be sustaining hope in the client who has been made redundant and who is now searching desperately for another job. Support may be a willingness on the part of the nurse to maintain the relationship, to resume contact whenever the client feels the need and for whatever purpose.

But support is not a permanent leaning post. If it were, the client may well be discouraged from establishing his own strengths. If it is a post on which the client leans, just as a young sapling may need a support until it becomes fully established, it must be gradually, and gently but firmly withdrawn as soon as he is sufficiently psychologically mature to stand on his own. Irreparable harm may be done to the client who has become overdependent on counselling support. If this happens, the motives and needs of the counsellor must be seriously questioned.

CHAPTER 7

EVALUATION

Just as evaluation, when using the nursing process, must influence reassessment and therefore further planning and delivery of care, evaluation of counselling brings about a reappraisal of the problem and of the areas for exploration. Evaluation, if undertaken with care and thought, can be an excellent learning device. If the client is an active partner in the evaluation exercise, both he and the nurse will be able to learn from each other. It may be less easy to state precisely what has been achieved in counselling than to demonstrate what has been achieved in the clinical care of patients. It may be easier for a patient who has been taught to manage a colostomy to be positive about his gains, than for Mr Link, who was helped to explore his feelings towards his son, or for Alan Driver, who was helped to reappraise his attitude towards work. Feelings cannot be excised when they cause problems, but very often being given permission and opportunity to talk about them will start the cleansing and healing process. But it may be some considerable time before the full benefits are realized.

On-going evaluation gives both nurse and client an opportunity to explore their feelings about what is happening and also to appraise, constructively, what should be done next. A terminal evaluation gives the client a feeling of completeness and also provides him and the nurse with an opportunity to look at some of those things which did not go according to plan, as well as those which did. An evaluation well carried out, not only looks backwards, it also looks forwards. It provides the client with something positive to carry with him into the future and the nurse with the satisfaction of a job completed.

Final evaluation

One of the first tasks is to carry out a review of what brought the nurse and the client together. It is possible, particularly when counselling has taken place over a period of time, that the original reason has faded into insignificance, as more recent and more momentous themes have been explored. In a way, it is like taking a journey: the traveller knows from where he has come, and knows roughly the route taken; but looking back, the starting point has become obscured, partly through distance, but also through time. Unlike taking a journey, however, it is often necessary for both client and nurse to look back in order to firmly establish the final position.

Start at the beginning

A useful place to start is the original contract. When Rachael and Alan felt that the time had come for Alan to go forward alone, they had a 'round table' session with the whole family. Rachael encouraged them to look back to the first day they met, and the problems of Alan's anxiety about work. Alan's remark, "I wasn't all that anxious, was I?" greatly amused the rest of the family. He genuinely could not remember how fraught things were. Rachael pointed out to them that just as events fade from the memory, so do feelings, particularly when some progress has been made towards resolving the problem. It is almost as if the prevailing mood and state of affairs has always existed. It may seem that asking the client to look back could cause a set-back; retracing one's steps may reveal obstacles that were previously hidden. This is true, and in a sense this criticism of evaluation is justified. But at the same time, it would not be the aim of evaluation to dwell overlong on any one issue. In a final evaluation, more emphasis should be placed on the way ahead than on what has taken place.

Alan told Rachael that when they met for the first time, he could not see how talking about things could help very much. "What I wanted was to get working again. When you began talking about my resentment, I couldn't see the point. When you left, I said to Ruth, 'I don't want to be psychoanalysed.' Ruth's reply was, 'Maybe that wouldn't be a bad thing, if it makes you easier to live with.' That really knocked me. I hadn't realized how difficult I had been. Neither had I realized just how self-pitying I was. So, I thought I would stick it out for the time we had agreed. You said you thought six sessions might be enough. After the second one, I began to see some light; and by the end of the six, when we started working on the action plan, things really did start to drop into place."

This was a very long speech from Alan, and Rachael felt pleased that he had voiced some of his early reservations which she had sensed but he had felt unable to reveal them.

The next stage in Rachael's evaluation was to look at the problems they had identified, then how they had been dealt with. This meant that they had to look at the goals and strategies adopted to reach them. Alan was pleased that so much progress had been made, except in the area of smoking. At this stage, Ruth intervened to say, "I think, darling, you have done marvellously. And I don't care any more if you smoke. I'd rather have a husband who smoked but had done so much with all those other things, than if you had not tried, and died on me." "This remark put it all into perspective", Rachael later commented to her mentor.

Positive growth

One of the things Rachael tried to do throughout the time with Alan was to encourage him, by pointing to areas of positive growth and to incidents that highlighted the gaining of insight. She did this at the time when there was movement from an attitude of nonacceptance to one of acceptance that his condition could be disabling. Another major victory (according to Alan) was when he mastered relaxation, something he now practised regularly. He avowed that this one technique had helped him live with his angina. He still maintained contact with the remedial therapist who was now working with him on a suitable exercise regimen.

While these areas of positive growth were being examined, Alan commented that in the early days of contact with Rachael he had suffered from "... some pretty foul moods of black despair. One of the things that really helped, was that you never once offered platitudes. So many people used to say, 'Oh, you'll be all right; everything will work out.' You never said that. It was the way you asked questions, as if you expected me to find my own answers, that gave me hope. Many times I felt as if I was drowning; then I would remember the tasks we had set; that spurred me on."

As Alan was talking, Rachael realized that here was another area of growth. He had never been one for 'this psychological stuff', but now he was talking at a feeling level.

Another positive area was that he had, of his own accord, written to the British Heart Foundation and suggested that, as there was no group locally, he would be prepared to help form one. This was still being explored. He said, "I shall have to watch it, though. I worked all hours God gave when I was in business; that must have had a lot to do with all this. I mustn't let the same thing happen." This was a salutary reminder and Rachael felt rewarded that there was so much evidence of an attitude change. Ruth's comment to Alan's remark was equally revealing. "But you don't have to, now. Then you were trying to prove something. We've got all we need. And you are a much happier man than you ever were."

The counselling relationship

Ruth's remark created a comfortable silence, catching every one up in it. Raymond apologetically said "Sorry to butt in; Mum's right. Dad's different and that means that we're different too. I thought he was really going to blow his top when I wanted to leave school. But then you gave us that job to do; that helped me to get things straight in my mind. Now I've decided to stay on and work for 'A' levels, if I get good 'O' level passes."

"We'll be sorry not to see you again, Rachael", Alan said. "Pop in when you're passing, any time, we'll be glad to see you. One of the things I've learned from you is to trust people. I was bitter—about life in general—when you came. Now I can honestly say that it has gone. I think that bitterness was making me believe that everyone was against me. You respected me and this helped me to respect myself and my capabilities. We don't know much about you, really, but we think you're lovely."

Rachael thanked Alan for his kind words and went on to say, "I've been wondering what I have got out of this contact with you all. Apart from the professional aspects, like a greater awareness of the resources and information available, I've learned a great deal about myself. You may not have realized it, but there were times when I went away feeling very discouraged, particularly when other people seemed so obstructive towards you. Quite often I felt like marching up to them and giving them a piece of my mind. It was difficult for me to sit back and let you get on with it—all on your own. So, I had to learn patience. There were times, too, when some of your questions and queries set bells ringing in my emotions. At one stage you said, 'I don't feel as if there is much to live for.' This really got me mad. It made me feel that I was wasting my time. My boss had to take me to task and as we talked round it, I could see that I wanted to be in control. I was very angry when she suggested this to me, and I stormed out of her office. But as I was driving away, I realized that I was gripping the wheel so tightly my knuckles were white. I said to myself, 'Rachael, you're afraid of losing control.' My boss was right. I wanted you to do what I thought you should do. That was a powerful lesson. Thank you. I had to learn what it was to go where you wanted to go and at your pace."

Success?

This case study has been chosen because it demonstrates some degree of success. But success is not always so easily measured. A person who comes for one session and leaves saying, "I feel better for having talked it over, even though there is nothing you can actually do", may then be more able to cope with life.

Angela, a middle-aged woman, came to a counsellor. She had multiple difficulties arising from a disastrous second marriage. She had left her first husband, "a boring and uninteresting man", for a "good looking, jolly, charming man", who later turned into a criminal and who, at the time she met the counsellor, was in prison. She poured out her story, saying as she finished, "I know there's nothing you can do. But it has helped to talk about it and not hide it."

Failure?

Roy was a youth counsellor. Andrew was one of his constant clients, never able to hold down a job. Roy spent many hours with him, and many times he helped him get jobs and with frequent regularity he appeared jobless for another chat. In one of his jobless periods, he stole a car, crashed it and was killed. Did Roy go wrong somewhere? Was there something he could have done? Some stop he could have pulled out? Some technique he could have used to prevent this tragedy? Success and progress or failure—whose responsibility is it? Whose credit or whose blame? Unlike the nurse carrying out a nursing procedure, the counsellor has no prescription to follow and ultimately it is the client who must shoulder the responsibility for his own decisions and actions. Andrew had a choice. Nothing 'made' him steal that car; it was his choice. It is certainly true that he may have cried loud and long for help and perhaps Roy did not hear him. When the news was broken to Roy, he was distressed to think that maybe he had not done all he could to help Andrew. This is a natural question to ask. It had the effect of making him stop and re-evaluate: that was positive and constructive. But for Roy to have taken on his shoulders the responsibility for Andrew's actions would have been taking an unfair burden and most certainly would seriously have affected his counselling.

The nurse, as counsellor, is in a similar position as when she is nursing a patient who refuses to take his medication. The choice is his, and must remain his. It is hard to stand by and do nothing when a patient, obviously in need of prescribed treatment, refuses to carry it out. But if the consequences of noncompliance are fully explained and understood by the patient, the nurse must then leave him to make the final decision.

Shared responsibility

The nurse can never remain absolutely neutral or unaffected by the outcome of counselling. It would be all too easy when counselling ends without seeing positive results to pass all the responsibility onto the client. If the nurse feels, "If only he had been more open, more communicative, less defensive", and so on, this should lead to her fully evaluating her own contribution. Similarly it may be easy, when counselling ends positively, for her to accept all the credit, forgetting that whatever her contribution has been, it was the client who was in focus throughout; and whatever was happening within her, much more was likely to be happening within the client. If she experienced growth from conflict within the counselling relationship, much more did the client experience conflict and subsequent growth. To him then must go the credit for whatever success has been achieved. Likewise, lack of success must remain with the client. The nurse as counsellor shares in both.

Finale

On pp. 50 and 57 reference was made to 'note taking'. For one's own professional development, some time should be devoted to making a summary of what has taken place throughout counselling. The model on which this book is based may be a useful structure for this summary. It is possible that what is included in the summary may never be read by any one other than the nurse herself. But the fact that she has taken time and effort to commit it to paper may, at some time in the future, be a useful resource for her, when pondering on a particular point in counselling. Experience can never be wiped out, but when experience is reinforced by evaluation, many of the interactions, the words, the nuances that so quickly fade from the memory, are captured in a way that experience by itself cannot do. If the nurse feels that the final evaluation is proving too difficult, that may be because evaluating her own part in the process is eluding her. It is possible, for example, that some aspect of the relationship between herself and the client is proving a stumbling block. If the stumbling block is not removed it will remain an obstacle in the way of effective counselling. Stumbling blocks can be turned into stepping stones by an honest and in-depth evaluation.

Sometimes one of the most difficult things to do, is to say 'good-bye'.

Summary of the Wessex model of counselling

Stage 1: Meeting the client
The counsellor and client begin to establish a relationship in which both feel that they are able to work together in an area which is causing concern to the client. It is at this stage that client and counsellor arrive at a contract which entails commitment from both of them.

Stage 2: Identify the problem
In this stage the client and counsellor identify the specific problem or clarify which particular problem needs to be, or could be, tackled first. It is at this stage that the client may need help to accept ownership of his problem.

Stage 3: Explore the problem
During this stage the client and counsellor explore the significant aspects of

the problem, the interaction between these aspects and how these interactions involve other people and other areas of the client's life. The general aim is for the client to increase his self-awareness and insights and to marshal these new strengths in working towards an action plan.

Stage 4: Action plan

The client can contemplate action only when he feels sufficiently free from the forces which have been restraining him and when he feels confident that he is able to use the inner resources which his new-found insights and awarenesses have released.

Stage 5: Implement the action plan

The client and counsellor may part company before this stage is reached, if the client feels he has the confidence to carry through the action plan without assistance from the counsellor. The client may need help to locate and use agencies which can provide information and assistance. He may need help to acquire new skills.

Stage 6: Evaluation

Evaluation should be on-going throughout counselling. When counselling is terminating, a complete evaluation is essential for both counsellor and client.

APPENDIX A

THE CITIZENS' ADVICE BUREAU SERVICE*

The aims of the Citizens' Advice Bureau are:

1. To ensure that individuals do not suffer through ignorance of their rights and responsibilities or of the service available; or through an inability to express their needs effectively.
2. To exercise a responsible influence on the development of social policies and services, both locally and nationally.

The service, therefore, provides—free to all individuals—an impartial service of information, guidance and support, and makes responsible use of the experience so gained.

The bureau service sees itself as the well-informed general practitioner of the social services, combining the roles of prevention, diagnosis and referral to the specialist consultants. It provides a friendly, nonstatutory service of advice and help. Any member of the public may walk into any Citizens' Advice Bureau and ask for help, information or advice. Help will be given to fill in a form, or explain a new piece of legislation and how it is likely to affect the inquirer's own circumstances. Staff will make telephone calls and draft letters. The bureau will stand between the inquirer and the organization, government department, authority or individual with whom he is at odds. The points of view of each is put to the other and this, in the majority of cases, results in a solution acceptable to both sides. A growing number of

---

*Prepared by the author from the booklet 'The Citizens' Advice Bureau Service'.

bureaux are becoming involved in tribunal assistance and in representation at County Courts. Specialist advice sessions, when solicitors or accountants, for example, deal with inquirers' problems, are organized.

The Citizens' Advice Bureau Service is made up of about 900 full- and part-time bureaux throughout the United Kingdom. Each bureau is a local self-governing unit, organized in a community for the citizens of that community. The day-to-day administration of a bureau is the responsibility of the bureau organizer. The staff may be paid or voluntáry, full or part time. Training—initial and on-going—is provided for all staff. Local authorities provide almost all the financial support in the form of grant aid. This does not influence the independent stance of the bureau serving the local community.

APPENDIX B

HOSPITAL INFORMATION UNIT*

Help for Health began in 1979 as a British Library project which investigated the need for information about the voluntary sector in health care. From this research it seemed that health-care staff were constantly seeking the addresses of self-help groups, details of the help provided by voluntary organizations or the educational literature produced by patient organizations, but had no readily available and accurate source of this information. The Help for Health Information Service was set up to answer these needs and is now funded by the Wessex Regional Health Authority. It is a unique service and forms the largest collection of self-help information in the United Kingdom.

Patients and disabled people in the community need information to enable them to understand their condition, to cope with it at home, and to make full use of the voluntary and statutory resources available to them. They may wish to use voluntary organizations for practical help with accommodation, transport, recreation, holidays, employment. With problems such as mastectomy, colostomy, spinal injury, bereavement, counselling by people who have gone through the same experience could be of great support to the patient. Help for Health is an information service which can alert patients, and health-care staff acting on their behalf, to voluntary organizations, self-help groups and publications to help them to understand and cope with health problems.

---

*Prepared by Robert Gann, Librarian. 'Help for Health', Wessex Regional Library Unit, Southampton General Hospital.

Help for Health is:

A resource centre with the addresses of over 2000 national and local patient organizations, many offering specialist counselling, and a major collection of patient-information materials, largely in book and leaflet form.

An inquiry service answering 300 inquiries a month from health-care staff, social workers, voluntary bodies, patients and members of the public. Inquiries are received by telephone, letter or in person. The service is staffed by a qualified librarian and a clerical officer.

A publisher producing information sheets, a newsletter and a series of guides to information on a variety of health problems.

Nurses, and in particular health visitors, regularly form the largest group of users of the Help for Health Information Service.

APPENDIX C

SOCIAL SERVICES WITHIN THE HOSPITAL*

The National Health Service Act of 1974 states that social work help should be available and accessible to patients and their families who themselves ask for help, or who are referred at any stage of their treatment.

To facilitate this service, hospital-based social workers are employed by the local authority social services department, thus providing the hospital patient and his family with direct access to the resources of the social services department. In addition, the patient will have a continuity of social worker as the support will continue from the health-based worker when the patient is discharged home where this is seen as necessary.

Social workers are based within the hospital so as to be active members of the multidisciplinary team, and to provide an overall assessment of the patient's total situation and to help plan for any needs the patient or his family may have, and to help ensure that the appropriate community resources are mobilized to ensure as successful a discharge home as possible.

The social services department thus offers the following broad range of resources:

1. A social-work service for personal and family counselling—especially where the patient and/or his family are having to adjust to

---

*Prepared by Ian Allured, Assistant Principal Officer (Health), Hampshire Social Services Department.

considerable changes in their normal functioning and personal circumstances, or where the illness is exacerbating existing problems.

2. A wide range of domiciliary and residential services.
3. Knowledge of statutory and voluntary resources within the community.
4. Experience and resources relating to the following main client groups: children; the elderly; the physically handicapped; the mentally ill; the mentally handicapped.

Most hospital social-work departments have a completely open referral system whereby referrals are welcome from any source, but as a matter of courtesy it helps if the patient is made aware of the referral and is in agreement with it.

The actual day-to-day running of social-work offices within hospitals may vary from authority to authority but the above general picture should act as a guide to the range of services available. If in doubt the hospital social work office or the local social services area office will be able to provide more specific information.

APPENDIX D

SOCIAL SECURITY MATTERS*

The nurse, from time to time, may encounter clients who are experiencing some difficulty over their state benefits. The notes pages of each allowance book answer many questions. More detailed advice can be obtained from the local Department of Health and Social Security (DHSS) office. The address of the issuing office should always be on the allowance book. Advice can always be obtained from the local DHSS office as well. If the nurse does not know their whereabouts, look them up in the local telephone directory under "Health and Social Security, Department of". They are open to the public 09.30 to 15.30 hours, Monday to Friday, but are available to answer telephone inquiries between 08.30 and 17.00 hours. It is not usually necessary to call in person at the office unless urgent advice or action is required.

The social security benefit system is complex—providing a range of benefits, some of which are dependent on National Insurance contributions; some are means-tested and some simply payable in particular situations, such as severe disability. Many people are not aware of their rights and may be missing out on help available. It would be impossible for the nurse to have full knowledge, but she may find it useful to carry with her (or have access to) two booklets, both of which are obtainable, free, from any DHSS office. These are 'Which Benefit?' and 'Help for Handicapped People'. They provide a brief guide to the benefits available in different situations such as disability, unemployment, etc., and will point out where to go for further guidance.

---

*Prepared by Mrs G. M. Kempster, Regional Information Officer, DHSS, London West Region, Basingstoke.

APPENDIX E

COMMUNITY HEALTH COUNCILS AND HOW TO USE THEM*

Community health councils were established by Parliament in 1974 to give the public a voice in the affairs of the National Health Service (NHS). A community health council may be thought of as the local public watchdog on NHS matters. Its services are funded by central government and are free to the users. A community health council—composed of 24 lay people—has three main roles:

1. To play a significant part when dramatic changes in services are undertaken. An example would be closure of a hospital.

2. To inform the public about the plans, ambitions and problems of the district health authority. On occasions it provides details on aspects of regional proposals and decisions.

3. To offer information, guidance and advice to people who experience difficulty in dealing with some issue related to the NHS.

In addition to offering advice on available services, where and how to use them, what standards are reasonable, or unreasonable to expect from the NHS, community health councils advise on the correct procedure when a member of the public wishes to complain about some aspect of the NHS.

---

*Summarized by the author from a statement prepared by: Mr Ken. M. Woods, Secretary, Southampton & S.W. Hampshire Community Health Council.

A person may make use of the information, guidance and advice offered by the community health council by contacting (by telephone, by letter or in person) the appropriate community health council office. The address may be found in the local telephone directory under the heading "Community Health Council".

The general aim is to ensure that every inquiry receives an answer from the most appropriate source, even though the inquiry or complaint concerns a department or organization other than the NHS.

Access to community health councils, which exist to ensure that members of the public receive the best possible service from the NHS, is informal and confidential.

APPENDIX F

A PROBLEM-SOLVING MODEL

Identify the problem

1. Is there a problem? if so, what is it precisely?
2. Who says there is a problem?
3. Who has the problem?
4. What other people are involved? How are they involved?
5. What is my role to be in helping ... resolve this problem? (Name the person or persons.)
6. What are my impressions of ...?
7. Why do I think and feel this way about them?
8. Any other points relevant to this stage?

Explore the problem

9. What areas does ... need help to explore?
10. How long has the problem existed?
11. What steps have been or could have been taken to resolve the problem?
12. Would (a) doing nothing (b) making changes create risks?
13. What changes are possible?
14. Which of (a) or (b) involve the greater risk?
15. What does ... have to (a) gain (b) lose?
16. What is the goal I think ... could work towards?
17. Any other points relevant to this stage?

Action plan

18. What action plan could I help ... draw up?
19. What steps could ... take to reach the goal set in 16?
20. Are there any changes I would (a) advise (b) advise against?
21. If any of the changes involve other people, what strategies can be devised to facilitate change?
22. What is my role in the action plan?
23. How will I know if change has taken place?
24. Are there any external factors which could work in favour of ... achieving his goal?
25. Are there any external factors which could work against ... achieving his goal?
26. Are there any internal factors which could work in favour of ... achieving his goal?
27. Are there any internal factors which could work against ... achieving his goal?

Evaluation

28. What question do I need to ask in an attempt to evaluate the problem-solving process?

This model may require some slight alteration according the client's specific circumstance or problem.

APPENDIX G

FORCE-FIELD ANALYSIS*

The client asks himself these questions:

1. What is the goal I want to reach?
2. What precisely is it that I want to achieve?
3. Is the goal realistic?
4. If it is not realistic, why not?
5. Can I identify some definite behaviour which needs to be changed?
6. If the behaviour involves someone else, what strategy can I devise to achieve this?
7. What effect will my goal-change have and on whom or on what?
8. How can I measure the change when it takes place?
9. When I have achieved my goal I shall be ...
10. When I have achieved my goal I shall do ...
11. The degree of risk in making a change is ...
12. The advantages of making a change are ...
13. The disadvantage of making a change are ...

Helping forces

14. Can I identify internal and external forces that would help me achieve my goal.

---

*Adapted from the original by the author.

EXAMPLES OF INTERNAL FORCES: Type of personality—optimistic, cheerful, outgoing, studious, caring, intelligent, thoughtful, intuitive, imaginative.
Age.
Health.

EXAMPLES OF EXTERNAL FORCES: Family, friends, locality, job, finance, housing, career, mobility, commitments, hobbies.

15. Can I identify internal and external forces that would work against me achieving my goal?

Any of the internal and external forces listed above may, in certain circumstances, act as restraining forces.

16. Which would be the easiest helping force to strengthen and work on to assist me to reach my goal?
17. Which would be the easiest restraining force to start diminishing its influence?
18. What strategy or strategies can I invent to achieve the aims in 16 and 17?

Repeat 16 and 17 as often as necessary with different forces.
The underlying principle is that by strengthening the helping forces and diminishing the restraining forces, a decision will be easier to make, because energy, which has been trapped by the restraining forces, has been released.

19. Have I achieved my goal?
20. Has my original goal changed in any way? How? Why?

APPENDIX H

COUNSELLING SKILLS LIBRARY

Holdsworth audio-visual, 18 Malbrook Rd, SW15 6UF

Tape 1   The counselling relationship

This deals with six basic counselling skills in establishing the counselling relationship: acceptance; empathy; genuineness; concreteness; confrontation; immediacy.

Very useful as a back-up for people who have had some counselling training to use on their own. Would be useful as an introduction.

Tape 2   The counselling interview

Discusses the short- and long-term aims of counselling; related to the wider issues of the educational role. The uniqueness of each counselling interview is stressed.

The four phases of the counselling interview are elaborated:

1. Negotiation.
2. Exploration.
3. Understanding the problem.
4. Planning ways of coping.

Tape 3   Personal counselling

This tape is not concerned specifically with education or with work although personal problems may be linked with both.

The discussion centres around four elements:

1. Information or lack of it and sources.
2. Difficulties in relationships.
3. Conflict within the client.
4. Underconfidence and anxiety.

This is applicable in many work situations and is related to case studies:

1. A teenage relationship problem.
2. Marriage guidance.

The analysis of the counselling process is particularly helpful.

Tape 4   Occupational counselling

Deals with the core skills of the counselling relationship and the framework of the counselling interview. Looks at choice, work effectiveness, work relationships and career development. Useful for any manager or supervisor with responsibility for staff.

Tape 5   Educational counselling

Any one who is asked for advice on educational matters—teachers, personnel officers, managers—would benefit from listening to the discussion. Learning problems are frequently linked to personal or interpersonal difficulties and also to occupational choices. Occupational goals may help to provide motivation to improve short-term effort.

Summary

These five tapes (each side runs for approximately 25 min) would provide a useful resource. They could be used by individuals in many settings. They could also be used in groups to stimulate discussion about counselling methods and problems.

BIBLIOGRAPHY

Argyle, M (1973) The Psychology of Interpersonal Behaviour, Penguin

Argyle, M (ed) (1981) Social Skills and Health, Methuen

Barclay, J R (1978) Foundations of Counselling Strategies, Kreiger

Berne, E (1964) Games People Play, Penguin

Bessell, R (1971) Interviewing and Counselling, Batsford

Beveridge, W E (1968) Problem Solving Interviews, Allen & Unwin

Biestek, F P (1961) The Casework Relationship, Allen & Unwin

Blum, L H (1972) Reading Between the Lines, International University Press

Borck, L E and Fawcett, S B (1982) Learning Counselling and Problem-Solving Skills, Haworth Press

Boy, A V and Pine, G J (1981) Client Centred Counselling, A Renewal, Allyn

Bradley, J C (1982) Communication in the Nursing Context, Prentice-Hall

Brammer, L M (1978) The Helping Relationship: Process and Skills, Prentice-Hall

Brown, D and Pedder, J (1979) Introduction to Psychotherapy, Tavistock

Burton, L (ed) (1974) Care of the Child Facing Death, Routledge and Kegan Paul

Byrne, P S and Long, B E L (1978) Doctors Talking to Patients, HMSO

Cavanagh, M E (1982) The Counselling Experience: Understanding and Living It, Brooks-Cole

Cronk, H M (1972) This Business of Dying, Nursing Times, 68 (31/8): 1100

Dean, H and Dean, M (1981) Counselling in a Troubled Society, Quartermaine

Egan, G (1975) Exercises in Helping Skills, Brooks-Cole

Foggo-Pays, E (1982) An Introductory Guide to Counselling, Ravenswood

Gilmore, S K (1973) The Counsellor in Training, Prentice-Hall

Grant, D (1979) The Physiotherapist as Patient Counsellor, Physiotherapist, July

Halmos, P (1977) The Faith of the Counsellor, Constable

Herron, J (1975) Six Categories Intervention Analysis, Guildford University

Katz, R L (1975) Empathy: Its Nature and Uses, Free Press of Glencoe

Keller, J F and Hughston, G (1980) Counselling the Elderly: A Systems Approach, Harper & Row

Kennedy, E (1977) On Becoming a Counsellor, Gill and Macmillan

Kennedy, E (1981) Crisis Counselling. The Essential Guide for Non-professional Counsellors, Continuum Press

Long, L, Paradise, L V and Long, T J (1981) Questioning: Skills for the Helping Process, Brooks-Cole

Maslow, A H (1971) The Farther Reaches of Human Nature, Eselan Institute

Menzies, I E P (1970) The Functions of Social Systems as A Defence Against Anxiety, Tavistock

Miller, S et al. Alive and Aware: Improving Communications in Relationships, Interpersonal Communications Programme Inc

Mitton, C L (ed) (1977) First Aid in Counselling, Attic Press

Morris, C (1965) Communication for Nurses, Littlefield

Morris, D (1978) Manwatching. Cape

Munro, E A, Manthei, R J and Small J J (1979) Counselling: A Skills Approach, Methuen

Nelson-Jones, R (1982) Theory and Practice of Counselling Psychology, Holt

Nierenburg, I and Calero, H H (1973) How to Read a Person Like a Book, Heinrich Hanau

Noland, R L (1978) Counselling Parents of the Mentally Retarded. A Source Book, Thomas

Nurse, G (1980) Counselling and the Nurse, HM&M

Nye, R D (1975) Three Views of Man, Brooks-Cole

Parry, R A (1975) A Guide to Counselling and Basic Psychotherapy, Churchill Livingstone

Poss, S (1981) Towards Death with Dignity, Allen & Unwin

Rogers, C (1950) Client Centred Therapy, H M Gousha

Rogers, C (1961) On Becoming a Person, H M Gousha

Smith, V M and Bass, T A (1982) Communication for the Health Care Team, Harper & Row

Stewart, W (1974) The Client Speaks, The Counsellor; Spring: 54–56

Stewart, W (1975) Nursing and Counselling: A Conflict of Roles? Nursing Mirror, 140: 71–73

Stewart, W (1979) Case Studies in Counselling, Occupational Health Journal, 31: 308–311, 568–578

Stewart, W (1980) Case Studies in Counselling, Occupational Health Journal, 32: 22–29, 76–83

Stewart, W (1982) Counselling and Organisational Development: Sameness and Difference, Counselling News, 39: 7–13

Truax, C B and Carkhuff, R R (1967) Towards Effective Counselling and Psychotherapy, Aldine Press

Tschudin, V (1982) Counselling Skills for Nurses, Baillière Tindall

Venables, E (1971) Counselling, National Marriage Guidance Council

Wallis, J H (1973) Personal Counselling, Allen and Unwin

Watts, A G (1977) Counselling and Work, Bedford Press

Wickes, F G (1977) The Inner World of Choice (A Jungian Approach to Psychotherapy), Coventure Ltd

Wiedenbach, E and Falls C E (1978) Comunication: The Key to Effective Nursing, Tiresias Press

INDEX